WORKING WITH FAMILIES
IN CRISIS
School-Based Intervention

The Guilford School Practitioner Series

EDITORS

STEPHEN N. ELLIOTT, Ph.D.
University of Wisconsin—Madison

JOSEPH C. WITT, Ph.D.
Louisiana State University, Baton Rouge

Academic Skills Problems: Direct Assessment and Intervention
EDWARD S. SHAPIRO

Curriculum-Based Measurement: Assessing Special Children
MARK R. SHINN (ED.)

Suicide Intervention in the Schools
SCOTT POLAND

Problems in Written Expression: Assessment and Remediation
SHARON BRADLEY-JOHNSON AND JUDI LUCAS-LESIAK

Individual and Group Counseling in Schools
STEWART EHLY AND RICHARD DUSTIN

School–Home Notes: Promoting Children's Classroom Success
MARY LOU KELLEY

Childhood Depression: School-Based Intervention
KEVIN D. STARK

Assessment for Early Intervention: Best Practices for Professionals
STEPHEN J. BAGNATO AND JOHN T. NEISWORTH

The Clinical Child Interview
JAN N. HUGHES AND DAVID B. BAKER

Working with Families in Crisis: School-Based Intervention
WILLIAM STEELE AND MELVYN RAIDER

WORKING WITH FAMILIES IN CRISIS
IN CRISIS
School-Based Intervention

WILLIAM STEELE, M.A., M.S.W.
*New Center Community Mental Health Center,
Detroit, Mich.*

MELVYN RAIDER, Ph.D.
Wayne State University

THE GUILFORD PRESS
New York   London

© 1991 The Guilford Press
A Division of Guilford Publications, Inc.
72 Spring Street, New York, NY 10012

Printed in the United States of America

This book is printed on acid-free paper.

Last digit is print number: 9 8 7 6 5 4 3 2 1

Library of Congress Cataloging-in-Publication Data

Steele, William.
   Working with families in crisis : school-based intervention /
William Steele, Melvyn Raider.
      212 p.   cm. — (The Guilford school practitioner series)
      Includes bibliographical references and index.
      ISBN 0-89862-362-6 (hardcover), — ISBN 0-89862-241-7 (paperback)
      1. Problem families—United States.   2. Family social work—United
States.   3. Crisis intervention (Psychiatry).   4. Personnel service
in education—United States.   I. Raider, Melvyn.   II. Title.
III. Series.
HV699.S68   1991
371.4′6—dc20   91-223
                                                                        CIP

About the Authors

William Steele, M.A., M.S.W., director of community services at New Center Community Mental Health Services, Detroit, Mich., is the author of several books on suicide prevention, trauma and loss in children, and developing crisis response teams in schools. He has over 25 years of experience managing family and youth crises and has trained over 20,000 school personnel. He has created and produced a number of nationally distributed educational videos on trauma and loss, including *Let's Stop Teen Suicide,* a 1986 Michigan Emmy winner. He is also the author of several school-based programs sponsored by foundations such as Hudson-Webber.

Melvyn Raider, Ph.D., is an associate professor of social work at Wayne State University, Detroit, Mich., where he specializes in courses on marriage and family therapy. He holds an M.S.W. from the University of Michigan and has clinical membership in the American Association of Marriage and Family Therapy. He is currently the director of a university-based research project examining the relationship between religion and the family.

Preface

Given the overwhelming array of problems that parents and children face today, it has become a virtual necessity to work with families in crisis within the school setting. Although the school's structure, resources, and responsibilities can limit involvement with families, brief intervention can be especially rewarding and beneficial to the student and his or her family.

This book attempts to provide a basic, practical, and applicable strategy for responding to families in crisis so as to prevent and/or minimize the self-defeating and even self-destructive behaviors that can emerge in students as a result of a family crisis.

The approach suggested is not intended to be clinical, but educational. Its focus is on immediate problem solving and restoration, when possible, of the family's level of functioning prior to the crisis. When successful the family will become better prepared for future crises and more able to prevent or reduce the psychological, social, emotional, and learning problems that can develop out of unresolved crises.

The tools presented here are easy to use and can yield a great deal of information and insight. The intervention process is presented in step-by-step stages which can be implemented immediately in a single family contact or used gradually over the course of several. The stages provide the worker with a structured, educational approach to intervention and empower the family with choices to help resolve the crisis themselves.

Working with families is not easy, but neither is it impossible nor unrewarding. We believe *Working with Families in Crisis* will provide the guidance and tools necessary to increase effectiveness in dealing with all types of family crises, and will allow the family to view the intervenor as credible, knowledgeable, and helpful.

ACKNOWLEDGMENTS

The authors wish to express their appreciation for the support, encouragement, advice, and long hours of editing Sue Sells devoted to this work.

In the preparation of this manuscript we had the valuable assistance of Jessie Kelly for whose secretarial help and sound suggestions we are grateful.

Too numerous to mention are the many families and educators whose willingness to share their experiences has proven not only invaluable but enlightening. Despite the sometimes negative image placed on schools, there are many caring, hard working, and committed educators who are making a significant difference in the lives of students and their families.

—WILLIAM STEELE
MELVYN RAIDER

Contents

I

FAMILY DYNAMICS

1

Family Crises Facing Schools

Working with families in crisis is not always rewarding. For example, the following scenario is common for school counselors who often have to deal with crisis situations. A student is in crisis, and the family has been called. Their response might be to refuse to come to school, to blame the school staff for the child's problem, to feel anger or indifference, or to agree to follow up on the recommendations and the referral that they have been given, but then fail to follow through once they leave the office. Such responses are not uncommon, and can make working with families challenging and often quite frustrating. Yet as difficult and complex as family intervention can be, when a crisis develops intervention must be attempted for the sake of the student.

Most educators will agree that 20 years ago there were fewer issues facing families, and that those issues that did arise were far less threatening and overwhelming than the issues currently facing the families of troubled students. Therefore, while more families are in crisis today, so too are the schools and personnel whose responsibility it is to attempt to help students and families resolve the family crises that directly affect the well being of these students. Given the increase in the number and depth of issues that can bring on a family crisis, this is a serious and often difficult responsibility.

The conditions that counselors and social workers must at times confront can seem overwhelming. This list provides samples of the situations that are indicative of crises facing families and schools (data from "Are We Pushing our Kids," 1986; "Bring Children Out," 1988; Centers for Disease Control [CDC], 1985; *Facts on Illiteracy*, 1988; Michigan Literacy; Rutter, Izard, & Read, 1986; Zinsmeister, 1990).

- Suicide is the third leading cause of death among young people in this country.
- Among 15–24-year-old white males suicide is the second leading cause of death.
- Among children under age 12 suicide is the eighth leading cause of death. In 1980 it was the tenth leading cause of death.
- In 1988, 2,000 minors were murdered—twice the number killed in 1965 when there were 6.5 million more people under age 18 in this country. Homicide is now the second leading cause of death among minors in the U.S.
- From 1983 to 1988 the number of minors arrested for murder increased by a startling 31%.
- The jump in murder arrests of children age 14 and younger was 28%.
- Seven million white children and 4 million black children under age 15 in the U.S. live below the poverty line.
- Half of all poor children grow up in households headed by women, and a quarter of poor black children live in homes where the mother has never married.
- Poor children are seven to eight times more likely to be the reported victims of child abuse and neglect than are children of middle or upper income families.
- More than 60% of all children born today will spend at least some time in a single parent household before reaching age 18.
- Nearly a quarter of all 19-year-old girls have had sexual intercourse before age 16. In 1984 the rate of illegitimate births among teenage girls was almost double that in 1980.

- There are an estimated 7 million latchkey kids under the age of 14 who are alone until their parents return from work.
- Today only one in five families with children is composed of a father as the "breadwinner" and a mother at home, compared with 41% 10 years ago.
- Two of four children age 13 and under live with parents who both work.
- The annual bill for 1 year of child rearing consumed 29% of the median family's budget in 1984, compared with 11% in 1966.
- At least 7 million children nationwide are cared for in family day-care homes or in child care centers. Seventy-five to ninety percent of family day-care facilities are unlicensed or unregistered.
- Working mothers spend an average of 11 minutes of quality time (defined as exclusive playing or teaching) with their kids during the weekdays and about 30 minutes per day on weekends. Fathers spend 8 and 14 minutes respectively.
- An estimated 1,300 step-families are formed everyday.
- One of the newer symptoms of school-age children today is the fear of failing.
- Fifty percent of American adults are unable to read an eighth-grade-level book.
- Forty-four percent of American adults do not read even one book in the course of a year.
- One child in six has tried marijuana and one in three alcohol before the ninth grade.

Suicide, violence, murder, sexual abuse, substance abuse, divorce, unemployment, poverty, illiteracy, teenage pregnancy, blended families, single parent families, families with two working parents and latchkey children—these are difficult issues for families, as well as for others who are responsible for the well being and learning of school-age children, to deal with. These issues are not, however, representative of all of the conditions or events that can precipitate a family crisis. There are many normal family tasks that can also create crises. Child rearing alone presents many potential hazards, each of which can result in a crisis (Scherz, 1971). Catastrophic events like fires, floods, and tornadoes can also bring about serious family crises.

The fact is that most families will face a major crisis of some kind, and the way in which a family responds to that crisis can determine how their children perform and relate in the school environment. This is very clear when families are exposed to violence. "Exposure to violence can cause deleterious effects on cognition including memory, school performance and learning. Significant alterations in personality are also repeated" (Pynoos & Nader, 1988, p. 456).

ELEMENTS OF A CRISIS

Who Defines a Crisis?

Experience might lead one to believe that the family facing a divorce is in far more of a crisis than the family in which both parents work and the children are either alone for several hours until their parents return home, or perhaps in which the parents' schedules are such that they are rarely together as a family. Each of these families, however, may perceive their situation to be a crisis and, in fact, each may present an array of serious problematic outcomes. The divorced family could actually perceive their situation to be an improvement, whereas the intact but working family might perceive themselves to be in crisis because of the conflicts that absences create for the entire family. How then is a family crisis defined?

From Change to Crisis

Any change, whether it be for better or for worse, creates stress. A promotion, for example, is a positive change. It is welcomed and appreciated, but it is also partially feared because of the many unknowns that can emerge from this change. There will be new information to process, new relationships to develop, new tasks to accomplish, and new decisions to make. Does such change necessarily lead to crisis? No, because when faced with change we can call upon past knowledge, relationships, memories, and coping skills to adjust to any new issues we are facing. Depending upon our past experiences and our coping skills we will either successfully meet the challenges of change or become overwhelmed by those challenges and experience a crisis. A family may be considered to be in crisis when that family faces an obstacle to important life goals that is, for a time, insurmountable through the utilization of customary methods of problem solving. A period of disorganization ensues, a period of upset, during which many abortive attempts at solutions are made (Caplan, 1964, pp. 40–41). Families that are in crisis have simply not been able to cope successfully with or adjust to the changes that have taken place within their family system.

Not an Event But a Perception

A family crisis is not necessarily an event, but rather a family's perception of an event as being dangerous or threatening, something they do not, cannot, or have not succeeded in resolving, removing, avoiding, or controlling. Understanding this helps to explain why two families can react so differently to the same event. Also, an event facing a family may pose a threat that is perceived as either real or impending. A family being held hostage by a crazed gunman faces a real threat, while a family fearing for the safety of its members because of changes in the neighborhood faces a more pending threat. There is no distinction, however, between real and pending if each is perceived by a family as a threat that they cannot manage.

Responding to a Threat

When families are unable to resolve the threat facing them they often move into a crisis state. This state is so intense that the family may desperately grab on to whatever promises to remove the intense fear and anxiety that are brought on by the threat they face. The family, for example, does not confront the drinking problems of one of its members because this would increase the possibility of a conflict that would be worse than the ongoing situation. A family that has experienced the suicide of one of its members may refuse to talk about that suicide among themselves because such talk creates too much pain for the survivors. In both of these examples the avoidance of confrontation is self-defeating. It places the families in jeopardy as opposed to helping them. Families may even recognize this yet continue the behavior. Why?

Self-defeating behaviors can be rewarding. When faced with the potential threat that is created by a member who has a serious drinking problem, a family's failure to confront that member can temporarily avoid both serious arguments and erratic behavior by the drinker. Avoidance temporarily removes the threat posed by this individual. Not talking about the suicide of a family member temporarily removes the threat of the overwhelming pain associated with that suicide, and therefore is also temporarily rewarding. Such behavior allows the rest of the family to feel safe again, to feel free from the anxiety and fear that accompany the threatening situation. What is critical to understand is that any behavior that reduces anxiety may become repetitious, even if it is self-defeating or self-destructive.

According to Warner (1966) there are six steps leading to the use and repetition of self-defeating behaviors.

First: Any reaction pattern that actually serves to reduce anxiety is a "rewarding" pattern as far as a person's emotional needs are concerned.

Second: We know, in line with basic learning theory, that any such "rewarding" pattern of response becomes "stamped in," and therefore persists. This agrees with common sense: We tend to repeat behavior that permits us to lower anxiety.

Third: A pattern of response may serve admirably to lower anxiety, but fail dismally regarding success in life. Obvious examples here are chronic alcoholism, drug addiction, and avoidance of work.

Fourth: When a pattern of response serves to reduce anxiety, then, in time, we crave to repeat that pattern.

Fifth: If this anxiety-reducing behavior happens to be self-defeating in regard to the individual's long term goals, this is unfortunate; but it does not at all preclude the repeated use of this self-defeating pattern in the individual's daily efforts toward maintaining freedom from anxiety.

Sixth: We know that various reaction patterns become fixed according to the degree to which they permit drive reduction—in this instance, anxiety reduction. Therefore, it follows that such self-defeating patterns are reinforced by the anxiety reduction which attends their use, and that such patterns tend to be self-perpetuating.

Another way to say it is this: Behavior may be *adjustive* without being *adaptive*. That is, behavior may permit anxiety reduction without in the least assisting the individual's long term welfare. It may even be seriously injurious to it. (pp. 172–173)

GOAL OF CRISIS INTERVENTION IN SCHOOLS

The goal of crisis intervention with families is to prevent self-defeating or self-destructive behaviors and to replace them with effective, adaptive coping skills that can reduce anxiety and enhance the family's ability to successfully manage this and future crises they may face, or at least return them to their level of functioning prior to the crisis state. There are several specific strategies for achieving the healthy resolution of a crisis that fall well within the parameters of school personnel (Steele, in press). Figure 1.1 provides an overview of the life of a crisis and intervention strategies appropriate for use in the school setting.

Normalizing the Experience

The family in crisis is not at all sure of what is happening or why. This factor, and the range of feelings associated with the crisis state, often leave the individual thinking that his or her reactions are not normal. This further compounds the fear

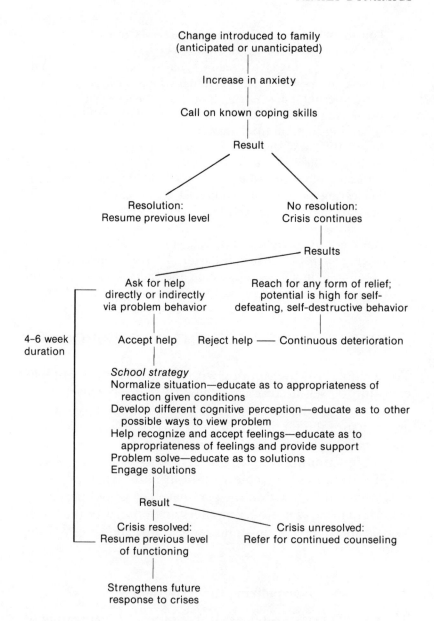

FIGURE 1.1. The life of a crisis.

that they are about to lose all control. Clarifying with the individual what the crisis state is and why it has occurred helps to normalize the experience, thereby reducing his or her level of anxiety. In other words, the family members need to understand that their feelings and behaviors are not unusual given the situation they face.

The family in crisis, for example, may feel hopeless and helpless. An understanding that these feelings are quite normal, given the current circumstances, can be very calming. Informing the family that while they may feel helpless, help is available, allows them to realize that their situation is not permanent. Normalizing the situation serves to reduce their level of anxiety, thereby allowing them to feel more in control. This, in turn, allows them to be able to become more focused on the possible steps they can take to reach healthy crisis resolution.

In a crisis a cognitive understanding of the obvious is sometimes lost. Explaining that being unsuccessful in resolving their crisis on their own does not mean that they will never be successful again can help the family in crisis to focus on resolution. Another example is that a failure to make things work does not mean they are a failure as a family. It only means that they have not had the information needed to know what else they might do. These seem quite obvious, but need to be explained if you want to help normalize the family's reaction to its crisis.

Different Cognitive Perception of the Situation

The previous goal focused on the developing of a different cognitive perception of a crisis as a normal reaction when the available coping skills and resources have failed to resolve the crisis. In this step, a different cognitive perception of the situation is focused on in order to help the family see the situation for what it is, no more and no less.

For example, the suicide of a friend who had expressed suicidal feelings does not mean that the friend to whom this was communicated is guilty of causing that suicide. In many such cases the children involved simply had never been taught that people who talk about killing themselves can be serious and that someone who can help must be told immediately. Once they are taught that those who talk about suicide sometimes do attempt it (different cognitive perception), they are more likely to seek help for such a person.

Another example would be a child who is told repeatedly that he or she is incapable of learning. This may not reflect reality. Given the right environment and understanding of the potential barriers to learning, anyone can learn. History is filled with volumes about successful individuals who were perceived to be incapable of learning or succeeding during their youthful years.

Therefore, a different cognitive perception of the situation may be achieved by exploring new information with family members, providing different perceptions of what is actually occurring in their situation, changing any negative, subjective interpretations that may have been received from others, and reviewing the possibilities or opportunities available to family members to resolve their crisis despite the conditions they face. A helpful cognitive response to any crisis is the attitude that conditions or situations do not determine what kind of family we are, the kind of family we are capable of being, or the kind of future we are capable of realizing. The only determining factor is how we choose to react to each condition or situation. This attitude explains how two families facing the very same conditions can respond so differently.

Recognition and Acceptance of Feelings

Distorted perceptions of a situation are due in part to distorted emotional reactions to the situation. Not until feelings are verbalized can the distortions be corrected and mastery over feelings be regained. In this sense, the feelings associated with the crisis state must first be recognized. Then the family can be encouraged to express those feelings in order to discharge the tension and clarify any distortions accompanying them. Only when this is accomplished can the family begin to regain mastery over those feelings that have hurled them into the crisis state.

Develop Problem-Solving Skills

The intent of crisis intervention is to help individuals resolve the crisis facing them. Problem solving is at the core of crisis intervention and is also a major function of school counselors.

WHY CRISIS INTERVENTION IN SCHOOLS?

The following are several key components related to the nature of a crisis that make the crisis intervention model appropriate in school settings.

Time Is Limited

A crisis is time limited. The state of active crisis will not last longer than four to six weeks (Golan, 1969; Hirschowitz, 1973). It either gets resolved through successful intervention or the family will engage in forms of denial, depression, projection, and other defenses, in addition to self-defeating or self-destructive behaviors in their attempts to alleviate fear. Without immediate help the risk of compounding their crisis with self-defeating problem-provoking behaviors is high. Because of the urgency felt by the family in crisis to feel safe again, it is imperative that intervention be provided as quickly as possible to prevent further deterioration. Crisis intervention, therefore, falls within the time constraints of the school staff.

Family Amenable to Help

The family that is experiencing pain is more likely to seek and accept help than a family that feels no pain (Rapoport, 1967). Fear is painful, anxiety is painful, and the experiencing of a threat is painful. In the face of such pain we feel vulnerable and are ready to do whatever has to be done to alleviate that pain. This makes families amenable to any immediate help that promises to remove the threat that is creating the pain they are experiencing. Schools can be invaluable in providing this help when it becomes obvious that a student is in crisis as a result of a family crisis.

Problem Solving

Crisis intervention relies heavily on problem solving and reeducation to help resolve the immediate crisis while preparing the family to better manage future crises (Steele, in press). The strategy itself is fairly consistent regardless of the crisis being presented, and can be effectively provided by trained school personnel. Therefore, it lends itself to the school environment. Keep in mind, though, that schools are not designated as clinical settings and so are not in the business of providing treatment. The problem-solving approach to crisis intervention, however, allows schools to remain within the boundaries of their responsibility to provide guidance, support, and opportunities to learn new ways of coping so as to stabilize the student.

Problem solving, when effective, not only helps families deal with immediate problem areas, but also teaches them a process they can turn to when faced with future crises (Pasewark & Albers, 1972). In addition, successfully negotiating their way through one crisis provides a family with the belief that as painful and as frightening as a crisis can be, they can work through it. This helps to reduce the intensity of the threat that may accompany future crises. Although the situation creating the crisis may not be able to be changed, effective education and problem solving will help the family to understand how that situation has threatened them (created their crisis) and to find ways they can effectively negotiate, avoid, or respond to that situation from an empowered position rather than a powerless position.

SUMMARY

Given limited community resources, long waiting lists, and the reluctance of families to engage in treatment, the crisis intervention approach is a nonthreatening alternative. It can be provided by schools, in a very limited time period, within the framework of reeducating both the student and his or her family to new ways or additional ways of approaching a difficult experience.

REFERENCES

Are we pushing our kids too hard? (1986, October 27). *U.S. News & World Report*, pp. 57–63.

Bring children out of the shadows. (1988, Spring). *Carnegie Quarterly, 33*(2).

Centers for Disease Control. (1985, March). *Report on suicide death rates.* Atlanta, GA: Author.

Caplan, G. (1964). *Principles of preventive psychiatry.* New York: Basic.

Facts on illiteracy in America. (1988). Syracuse, NY: Literacy Volunteers of America.

Golan, N. (1969, July). When is a client in crisis? *Social Casework,* pp. 389–394.

Hirschowitz, R. G. (1973, December). Crisis theory: A formulation. *Psychiatric Annals, 3,* 38–47.

Michigan Literacy, Inc. (Available from The Library of Michigan, P.O. Box 3007, Lansing, MI 48909.)

Pasewark, R. A., & Albers, D. A. (1972, March). Crisis intervention: A theory in search of a plan. *Social Work,* pp. 70–77.

Pynoos, R. S., & Nader, K. (1988). Psychological first aid and treatment approach to children exposed to community violence: Research implications. *Journal of Traumatic Stress, 2,* 445–472.

Rapoport, L. (1967, March). Crisis oriented short term casework. *Social Service Review,* pp. 38–41.

Rutter, M., Izard, C. E., & Read, P. B. (Eds.). (1986). *Depression in young people.* New York: Guilford Press.

Scherz, F. H. (1971, June). Maturational crisis and parent–child interaction. *Social Casework, 52,* 362–369.

Steele, W. (in press). *Developing crisis response teams in schools.* Holmes, FL: Learning Publications.

Warner, S. J. (1966). *Self-realization and self-defeat.* New York: Grove Press.

Zinsmeister, K. (1990, June). Growing up scared. *Atlantic Monthly,* pp. 49–66.

2

The Family as a System

Just as crisis intervention provides a workable framework for the school setting, family systems theory provides a workable model for understanding how families operate. It is necessary to have a basic understanding of how families operate before further exploring how crisis intervention works with families. Chapter 2 examines family systems and their key components. These will become the focus of intervention in the school setting.

We begin with a question. Why is it that parents often remove their child from counseling just at the point when progress is being made in bringing about a necessary and beneficial change in the child's life? When we view the family as a system we see that any change in one of its members, whether it be negative or positive, creates a new set of changes, challenges, choices, and sometimes crises for the other members of that system. If those changes significantly threaten other members (create a crisis) the members may attempt to block any further growth.

Families are repeatedly challenged to change. Over time roles must be altered, alliances shifted, and patterns of behavior adjusted. As old and comfortable ways of coping become useless, new ways must be discovered. Not everyone accepts change, and in fact, many fear it. Depending upon a person's level of confidence, sense of empowerment, and previous experiences with something new, any change may be vehemently resisted. Family systems are no different in their responses. Closed family systems resist many types of change, but open family systems, because of their experiences, may be nervous or cautious about change, but eventually adapt.

Approaching the family as a system when a crisis is presented, can, given the limited time available in a school setting, increase the effectiveness of the intervention provided on behalf of the student. The following is a brief description of the structures, boundaries, and processes that make up such a system.

A family system is made up of subsystems that are interdependent and interactive. The subsystems are the individual family members who interact with each other and thereby establish relationships. The basis for the relationships may be utilitarian (such as economic, legal, or physical) and/or socio-emotional (Sedgwick, 1981).

In Figure 2.1 the circle represents the overall family system, while each "I" represents a subsystem or individual within the system. As is illustrated, each individual interacts with one another. Different pairs, triads, or groups will also have different influences on these relationships. For instance, between parents economic issues may have a greater influence on their relationship (subsystem) than they would have on a relationship between father and son. A mother–daughter relationship may have different emotional influences than a brother–sister relationship. The physical influence between father and daughter may be different than between father and son.

FAMILY SUBSYSTEMS

In Figure 2.2 the lines of interaction between individuals demonstrate that each member has a connection to every other member. These connections may be strong or weak, but

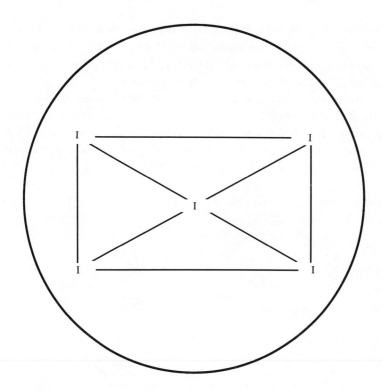

FIGURE 2.1. Family subsystem. "I" represents interacting subsystems or individuals.

they always exist. The lines change, but patterns develop over time. A son's connection to his mother may have stronger emotional ties than his connection to his father, although in different situations this can change, depending upon the roles of the parents and their actual involvement with their child.

This is not new information, but it can provide a valuable framework when working with families at a time of crisis. A simple exercise that can teach the intervenor as well as the family members a great deal about their particular family system is to have each member depict all of the members within a circle. They then identify the members (i.e., mom, dad, brother, sister). Using a solid line they then connect themselves to the member to whom they presently feel closest. A broken line is used to depict the relationship with the member whom they feel the furthest from.

Following this, each member's drawing is presented one at a time. Each member is asked if he or she agrees or sees the relationships differently and if there are any surprises. Each member can then be asked to explain what specific behaviors create a solid or a broken connection. A son may show a solid line connection to mom and a broken line to dad. His explanation could be as simple as mom is around the house more than dad.

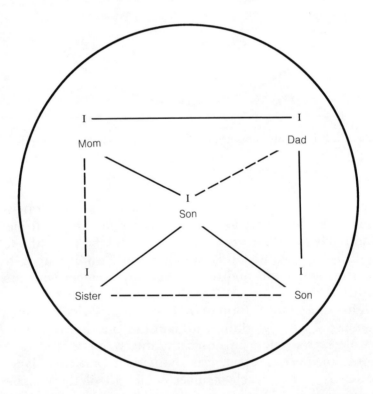

FIGURE 2.2. Subsystem relationships. Solid lines are strong relationships. Broken lines are weak relationships.

This exercise can help to define the subsystem's relationships and dynamics, while at the same time help to identify what changes might help to stabilize the family. An obvious question in this regard is whether these patterns existed prior to the crisis or changed as a result of the crisis. If they have not changed, one might interpret this to mean that the crisis has not altered the actual system, and that an alteration in these relationships has not created the crisis.

Boundaries

The family system is separated from other systems by boundaries. These boundaries serve to sort out, accept, or reject information that comes into or flows out of the family system. "Boundaries that surround the family are social (norms, expectations, myths), physical (space, territory, housing), emotional (feelings), historical (legacy, belief, expectation), and individual (ability, need, desire)" (Sedgwick, 1981, p. 13). The family is also bounded by its beliefs, morals, and values. These beliefs are the bases for the formal and informal rules and norms that the family establishes to guide its members in the ways they behave toward each other, other people, and toward the groups that comprise other systems in the environment. Boundaries evolve as a function of family history, social contact with others, and religious values.

Family morals and values and religious morals and values often become intertwined. Hines and Boyd–Franklin suggest that the values of many Black Baptist families are directly or indirectly derived from religious doctrine (McGoldrick, Pearce, & Giordana, 1982, p. 96). Similarly, among Fundamentalist Protestants, Christian religious values serve as the major frame of reference for determining family values and ethical positions. (For example, love is viewed as the possession of the qualities of devotion and loyalty.) Establishing a family is also at the core of the Jewish tradition. Their belief in the importance of the family as a sacred institution stems from the idea that it is a violation of God's law not to marry.

Religion is also a powerful determinant of the nature of the boundaries between families and others in their environment.

According to McGoldrick, Pearce, and Giordano, Fundamentalist Christian families may establish boundaries between themselves and outsiders by projecting fear and hostilities on outsiders in the form of scapegoating. Jewish families have historically established boundaries between themselves and non-Jews by actively discouraging intermarriage. Intermarriage was perceived to be a threat to the survival of the Jewish people and a violation of a major family value that had been derived from traditional religious documents (McGoldrick, Pearce, & Giordano, 1982).

In Figure 2.3 we see the family system. The outer circle represents the various boundaries. We briefly described the influence of religious boundaries as an example of the influence such boundaries have on family responses. Other boundaries, as indicated earlier, can include a variety of different

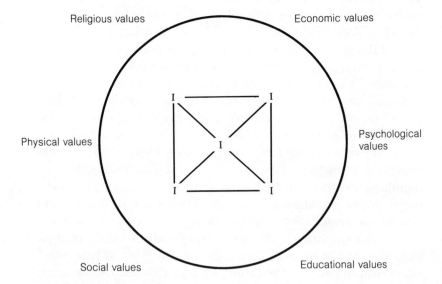

FIGURE 2.3. Family boundaries. The outer circle represents systems boundaries.

factors. The physical boundaries of the suburbs will reflect different influences than those of the city. Economic boundaries certainly limit or expand family opportunities.

When working with families it is sometimes helpful to have them define for themselves the boundaries that exist that are both helping and hindering them as a family during their crisis. Simply asking them what their beliefs are about mental health centers or psychiatric facilities (psychological values) can quickly establish whether their beliefs will be a deterrent or an aid. By helping families to focus on beliefs related to specific boundaries we can sometimes more clearly define the frustration, hopelessness, anxiety, and vulnerability experienced during a crisis.

The most obvious question related to boundaries concerns both the family's expectations of what intervention can accomplish, and their beliefs about involving others in the intervention. One of the more helpful interventions with families in crisis is the involvement of extended family members or friends as supports. When a mother, for example, is unable emotionally to care for her child during crisis, an aunt, grandmother, or even a friend can temporarily care for the child while mom stabilizes. If that mother, however, believes that any such help is a sign of weakness or failure (psychological value), the crisis resolution is going to be far more difficult to achieve.

Family Processes

Family processes, which are related to assessment and intervention, must be identified. Given the limited amount of time that schools are likely to be involved in family crisis intervention, family processes may be even more important in this setting than family structure and boundaries. This is the area in which a great deal of problem solving can take place, as well as a reeducation about the reasons for the crisis they are experiencing.

Family systems involve processes that taken together determine the pattern by which the family organizes communication and interaction among the family subsystems. Family processes regulate how the family assimilates information, makes decisions, resolves conflict, facilitates individuation, provides socio-economic support, accommodates stress, and responds to change. These family processes or system linkages are identified as emotional bonding, decision making, information processing, conflict resolution, and communication. An example of the way in which they might relate in an actual family can be seen in Figure 2.4.

Emotional bonding is the amount of both depth of feeling and breadth of attachment among the family members. Positive emotional bonding, such as loving and caring, provides a sense of connectedness that brings the family together. Helen Harris Perlman describes this quality as "a human being's

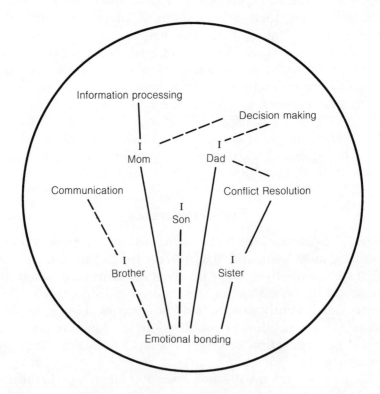

FIGURE 2.4. Family process. Solid lines reflect strong process skills. Broken lines reflect weak process skills.

feeling or sense of emotional bonding with another. It leaps into being like an electric current or it emerges and develops cautiously when emotion is aroused by and invested in someone or something and that something or someone connects back responsively" (Perlman, 1979, p. 15). This relationship allows a family "to feel secure and thus to go forward to risk new learning and new experiences. It combines a warm acceptance of each person in his/her specialness and his/her present being" (Perlman, 1979, p. 30). Emotional bonding also influences the quality of the sexual relationship between the husband and wife.

Information processing refers to the patterns of information utilization. Effective information processing combines the use of both information from within the family as well as information from community sources such as neighbors, physician, school teacher, or pastor. Beavers suggests that effective information processing is based on a framework where knowledge is viewed as limited and finite, and in which the family never possesses unchangeable truth (Beavers, 1985).

Decision making is the process of choosing among alternatives. This should result in a choice that is consistent with the family member's age, experience, resources, and ability. Effective decision making is a process that seeks a balance between rigidity and diffuseness, and involves systemic openness. Ineffective decision making is characterized by family rules and myths that deny uncertainty.

Conflict resolution is the process of managing differences. Effective conflict resolution accepts that harmony is not necessarily always healthy. Differences are tolerated as each individual in the family changes and grows. Disagreements are handled openly rather than smoothed over or ignored.

Communication is the process in which words, actions, and gestures are used by each family member to share information and express his or her opinions, feelings, and personal desires. Effective communication involves skills in verbal expression, active listening, and in the negotiation of solutions to problems. Effective communication also involves the ability of each family member to clearly define their own wishes and needs.

CLOSED, OPEN, AND RANDOM SYSTEMS

Kantor and Lehr (1975) have developed an empirically based typology of the forms that families use to shape their processes. They have designated three basic types: closed, open, and random (see Table 2.1). In the closed family system, processes that produce stability are relied upon as reference points for order and change. In the open family system, order and change are expected to result from the interaction of relatively stable evolving family processes. In the random system, unstable process are experimented with as reference points for order and change (Kantor & Lehr, 1975).

Goal of Closed Systems

The primary goal of the closed type family is stability in all family processes. According to Kantor and Lehr durability, fidelity, and sincerity are the closed type family ideals in the "affect dimension," which refers to intimacy and nurturance. Family loyalties are valued above those of friends. Affection is composed with the emphasis on an enduring sense of belonging. In the power domain authority and discipline predominate. The power domain refers to the freedom to decide what each member wants. Rules are extensive and clear. Obedience does not mean submission, but rather an apprenticeship to something bigger than the self. In the meaning domain the closed type family strives to maintain a stable identity. The meaning domain refers to the family's explanation of reality and how it defines each member's identity. Their beliefs and values give family members a great deal of certainty about the world. Judgments and decisions are made based on a traditional ideological system (Kantor & Lehr, 1975).

Goal of Open Systems

The primary goal of the open type family is to create a family environment that is adaptive to the needs of both the individual members and family as a whole. According to Kantor and Lehr responsiveness, authenticity, and the legitimacy of flexi-

TABLE 2.1. Family System Characteristics

Area of assessment	Closed	Open	Random
1. Rule:	Authoritarian	Participatory	Random, anybody
2. Focus:	Family image of unity even if unity does not exist	Individual needs and family unity	Individual desires chosen over family unity
3. Affection: (Emotional bondings)	Covert	Overt	Overt and covert
4. Goal:	Stability	Flexibility	Spontaneity, exploration tolerated–encouraged
5. Ambiguity:	Not tolerated	Tolerated until clarity reached	Tolerated–encouraged
6. Conflict:	Not tolerated	Seen as healthy process	Inconsistent
7. Decision making:	Autocratic	Family participation	Individualistic
8. Information processing:	One-way (top-down)	Three-way (top-down, down-up, and across)	Random, inconsistent
9. Communication:	Secretive, restrictive pattern	Open, sharing, listening, negotiating patterns	Informal, from closed to open pattern
10. In a crisis:	Rigid, unyielding; creates greater vulnerability and potential for further deterioration	Yielding, flexible; open to help minimizing vulnerability and risk of continued deterioration	Lacks sufficient consistency; leaves it vulnerable but not at as great a risk as the closed system due to its tolerance for ambiguity

bility in expressing honest feelings are the affect goals of the open type family. Emotions are more overtly expressed than in the closed type family. Nurturance and intimacy, which enable the family to adapt, are sought. In the power domain complete family member participation in decision making assures that all members are heard. Persuasion rather than coercion is the open type family's mandate. Opposition is accepted and worked through as the family seeks the resolution of its problems. In the meaning domain the open type family values authenticity. Relevance, affinity, and tolerance are its goals. Its reasoning process progresses from a rational frame of reference. Argument and debate are viewed as mechanisms to reduce conflicting evidence so that as complete a view of reality as is possible will be obtained (Kantor & Lehr, 1975).

Goal of Random Type System

The primary goal of the random type family is exploration. Unlike the closed family, the random type family accepts nonuniversal answers. According to Kantor and Lehr, exploratory nurturance and intimacy are this type of family's goals in the affect domain. Emotions are variable and may reflect intensity at both ends of the emotional spectrum. The emphasis is on spontaneity, novelty, and humor. In the power domain individual choice is the norm. Rules are relaxed and relationships are informal. Interchangeability, free choice, and challenge rather than unity are the ideals. In the meaning domain all points of view are possible. Ambiguity is permitted and even encouraged as a representation of the perplexity and diversity of life. Creativity is valued and encouraged (Kantor & Lehr, 1975).

Family System Equilibrium or Integration

Equilibrium refers to a state of balance among system components or subsystems. Equilibrium is achieved when the members of the family are comfortable and secure with both the nature of the interaction among the subsystem components, and with the type and quality of the exchanges within the larger network of systems. Stability occurs when there is a commitment to a set of shared expectations. When such a commitment exists the energies of the family members become available for other things.

Equilibrium or stabilization is the overall goal of crisis intervention. Returning the family to its level of functioning prior to the crisis, or helping them to reach a more adaptive level of functioning as a result of the crisis, is the major objective. Not all families can or will reach new adaptive levels, and so simply returning them to the life they lived prior to the crisis may be a worthwhile endeavor, especially when compared to the deterioration and development of the self-defeating, even self-destructive, patterns that can emerge as a result of a crisis that goes unattended or unassisted by intervention.

SUMMARY

Approaching families in crisis from a systems viewpoint has several advantages. Being able to determine whether a family is closed, open, or random allows the intervenor to focus on the primary goal of each system in order to stabilize that system. Talking flexibility to a closed system family whose focus is on stability will be met with a great deal of resistance. Knowing the kind of system a family engages also allows the intervenor to more realistically define expectations and goals. Closed families are by far the most difficult to work with because of their intolerance for uncertainty and change. This fact does not negate the positive outcomes possible through crisis intervention, but it does better clarify those possibilities.

Each type of family will use certain processes more adaptively than others. Open families, for example, will engage all members in the decision making process. Closed families use more of an authoritarian approach, with decisions being made with little or no family involvement. In a crisis situation the open family process could actually make matters worse if the situation demands immediate action. (Whereas one person taking charge, i.e., the closed family response, might be the most adaptive response.) Understanding these processes as they relate to the different systems allows the intervenor to identify and reinforce those processes that are most beneficial in a crisis situation.

The following discussions of assessment and intervention will further define the use of systems information in the school setting. The focus will be on brief assessment and intervention strategies designed to help families with their crisis so that their child can maximize his or her learning potential in the school environment. Before addressing assessment and intervention, however, it is important to understand both the types of situations that can precipitate a crisis, and those coping skills that are either adaptive or maladaptive. In Chapter 3 we identify four crisis categories pertinent to families, and discuss adaptive and maladaptive coping skills and their relationship to family processes and system types.

REFERENCES

Beavers, W. R. (1985). *Successful marriage.* New York: W. W. Norton.

Kantor, D., & Lehr, W. (1975). *Toward a theory of family process.* San Francisco: Jossey-Bass.

McGoldrick, M., Pearce, J., & Giordano, J. (Eds.). (1982). *Ethnicity and family therapy.* New York: Guilford Press.

Perlman, H. (1979). *Relationship.* Chicago: University of Chicago Press.

Sedgwick, R. (1981). *Family mental health.* St. Louis: C. V. Mosby.

3

Families in Crisis

What are the crises that families face? How do crises differ? What family system adapts best to a crisis? What family system struggles the most when threatened by a crisis? Does this depend upon the type of situation that precipitates the crisis state? Is there a set of characteristics that identify the adaptive versus the maladaptive family response?

In this chapter we examine these questions as a means of arriving at a clearer understanding of the family characteristics that are most likely to lead to adaptive resolution, as well as those likely to result in maladaptive resolution. The vulnerabilities of family systems that invite crisis situations are also defined and discussed. It is important to understand system vulnerability in order to better prepare a system to utilize adaptive coping skills, which can be effective despite these vulnerabilities.

TYPES OF FAMILY CRISES

Caplan identified crises as both those events precipitated by everyday living and those created by hazardous events. Everyday events would involve the development stages of a family and its members (i.e., the birth of a child, first year of school, marriage of a child, retirement, and so forth). Hazardous events might involve serious illnesses, accidents, the need to move, and/or catastrophic situations like a flood or a fire. Every family faces anticipated developmental crises and most families face some hazardous situations, although these are less predictable (Caplan, 1964).

Extrafamilial–Intrafamilial

Hill describes similar categories. His extrafamilial and intrafamilial crises are similar to the hazardous and everyday living crises described by Caplan. Extrafamilial refers to those major hazardous events that happen outside of the family and are not under their control, such as economic recession, massive flooding, or a plane crash. Intrafamilial crises are those events that take place within the family, such as physical/sexual abuse, abandonment, substance abuse, suicide, teen pregnancy, or divorce. Again, most families, regardless of their system type, will be vulnerable to extrafamilial and intrafamilial crises, with the former events being less predictable (Hill, 1958).

Dismemberment

We view Pasewark and Albers' (1972) discussion of Eliot's delineation of the events that characterize family life most helpful. Dismemberment describes the loss of any member of the family, whether by violence, nonviolent death, abandonment, or simply the natural process of a child growing up and moving out of the home. Illness is also included here if the illness takes a member away from the home (i.e., via hospitalization). Any member loss, therefore, can become a potential crisis. This is understandable when we view the family as a system. If a mother takes ill and must be hospitalized, even for a brief period, the system loses its balance and will be faced with many "adjustment" choices. If the family is rigid and not used to change, or simply unable to be flexible, a crisis will result.

Ascension

Ascension is simply the opposite of dismemberment. It refers to the addition of a member to the family. Eliot (in Pasewark & Albers, 1972) specifically refers to the unplanned addition, but even an anticipated ascension, such as the desired addition of a newborn, makes for some difficult adjustments. Unplanned additions, of course, are more difficult to adapt to, if only because enough time has not usually been available for the other members to discuss and define how their lives, roles, responsibilities will have to change. Just remember how a class often reacts when a new student is added and you can understand how ascension can create a crisis for families.

Demoralization

Demoralization focuses on an unwanted behavior or condition of one of the family members. The family does not change in size, but one of its members creates a crisis by bringing about an undesirable situation, such as alcoholism, abuse, an extra marital affair, problem behavior, or an emotional disturbance. The key word is "undesirable," which is clearly defined by the family's perception of what is undesirable, or of what they will or will not tolerate. Unemployment is certainly not desired, but is likely to be more acceptable, for example, than the incorrigible behavior of a child.

Demoralization and Dismemberment/Ascension

The final category is demoralization accompanied by dismemberment or ascension. Suicide is both demoralizing and causes a disorganization of the system because of the absence of the deceased. Psychiatric hospitalization is also demoralizing and a "dismemberment" of the family. A grandmother diagnosed with terminal cancer is demoralizing, and her "ascension" by her coming to live her final days with the family precipitates many changes and the likelihood of a crisis.

All family systems are vulnerable and will likely experience all four of these types of crises. The nature of the system will predicate how well each crisis is resolved.

ADAPTIVE VS. MALADAPTIVE COPING

Caplan (1964), Hill (1958), Pasewark and Albers (1972), Rapoport (1962), Rooney (1958), and Steele (in press) present the characteristics of the family responses most likely to result in the successful resolution of a crisis and thereby prevent the maladaptive behaviors that can result from a poorly managed crisis. As these are reviewed it will become apparent that closed family systems, in general, present the least adaptive approaches. This is not to say that closed family systems cannot resolve crises, but only that adaptive resolution can be far more difficult for them to achieve.

The following are several of the key characteristics particular to adaptive coping, with their contrasting characteristics described below. Note that these characteristics are similar to those in open family systems. Also, the characteristics of each system often relate to the processes within that system (i.e., decision making, as discussed in Chapter 2).

Flexibility

The ability to bend and sway in a wind storm prevents trees from breaking in half. It is not size that makes the difference, but rather the degree of flexibility, or the extent to which the trunk can bend and deflect the storm without breaking, that determines its survival. Those that stand rigid and move little break the easiest.

Families are no different. Those that survive are flexible, not rigid. They can bend the rules and sway with the crisis, whereas those that hold a rigid stance often split apart. Flexible families will seek help, try out new situations, temporarily alter their routines, roles, and responsibilities, lower their expectations, and change their priorities. Rigid families, on the other hand, will not welcome change, will hold even tighter to their normal routine, will not accept help or outside resources, and will not change their priorities. These families may even increase their expectations. Rigid families simply do not bend and by not bending become very vulnerable.

Affection

To deal with a crisis alone is not only difficult. It limits successful resolution. Affection (emotional bonding) is a key to maintaining a sense of security, safety, and confidence during a crisis situation. For example, families that experience the suicide of one of their members (dismemberment and demoralization) are generally thrown into a crisis. Survivors often report that what they remember the most, and what meant the most to them at the memorial service for their lost loved one, was the number of people in attendance. They remember little of what was said, but do remember the show of affection they received through the presence of others.

The more rigid and inflexible the family, the less there will be any expressed affection. Anger, withdrawal, silence, and other forms of panic are more visible than any affection or support for one another. To be able to give affection to others when faced with a crisis projects hope and the belief that despite the present conditions things will be resolved. There is mutual trust, and a belief that "together we will work this out," as opposed to the more rigid response of "Don't touch me. Don't get close. Leave me alone, I'll handle this myself."

Physical and verbal expressions of affection during a crisis proclaim a family's united stance against that crisis. They allow the family members to draw strength from one another, and in so doing reduce the level of anxiety. In the face of a serious threat this unity allows them to be more "proactive" and less "reactive" in their responses.

Healthy Adult Relationship

Two parent families, with a husband and wife who trust one another, openly communicate, do not fear conflict, and are able to adjust their roles and responsibilities temporarily when one or the other is in the process of change or facing a crisis, are usually going to be successful at resolving a crisis. If the relationship is unsettled, filled with unresolved conflict, poor communication, and questionable trust, a crisis is only going to intensify these reactions.

We often hear it said that it takes a major crisis to draw people together. While we grant that a crisis provides an opportunity to learn and grow, it is still true that a poor parental relationship presents a major challenge at a time of crisis. If the foundations of trust, communication, and affection are fragile, a crisis is more likely to tear the couple further apart. Intervention can help, but will be limited simply because the foundation of the relationship is weak. These are the situations that often demand more of a long term approach outside the school setting. Crisis intervention may prevent further deterioration, but until the basic relationship issues are worked out this family will remain at risk. "At risk" families, for example, will frequently present a theme of separation, divorce, and/or abandonment. During a crisis this theme intensifies tremendously, and often appears to be the only option available. This is similar to a closed system response. Open family systems are not immune to divorce or separation, but this is generally not a major threat to open families. If a divorce actually takes place it usually comes after mature but unsuccessful attempts to resolve the issues.

In single parent families the same closed or open characteristics may exist between parent and child and/or between other adults. Contrary to popular opinion, single parents can and often do manage well, even in a crisis. It is not always easy, but if the single parent is flexible, open, accepting of support, and involved in healthy, supportive relationships with other adults, they will generally do well.

Healthy Parent-Child Relationship

The issues between parent-parent and parent-child are similar when one is determining the likelihood of a successful crisis resolution. Trust, affection, open communication, and flexibility must be there if resolution is to be successful. The children must certainly not be in fear of rejection, separation, or abandonment (neglect) by their parent. This will help to keep their anxiety in a crisis manageable.

The one differentiating factor between open and closed parent–child relationships is the unconditional love that the child experiences in the open system, as opposed to the much more conditional response from the parents in closed systems. Open systems place more emphasis on the importance of playing with the children, and letting them know beyond a doubt that their parents enjoy being with them. Parents may focus on the importance of achievement, but this is usually secondary to a mutually enjoyable relationship. Closed families often focus on achievement as an indicator of the child's love for the parent. A great deal of pressure can be exerted on the children to achieve, to the point where the relationships are only "favorable" when goals or expectations are being met. Achieving, therefore, becomes a "condition" of love.

Decision Making

In closed families decisions are made by the person in authority. "Ask your mother. She makes the decisions around here," is a typical response in closed families. Open families involve all of the members, when appropriate, in the decision-making process. Children have the ability to negotiate. In closed families children are told what they will do and how, when, and where they will do it. They have no say, no self-determination. After the death of a family member, for example, one person will emerge from a closed family and make all of the decisions regarding the service, burial arrangements, and the family adjustments that will have to be made. In open families a child's wishes would be elicited and respected.

Social Activities

Just as all of the members of an open system are appropriately involved in the decision-making process, they are also involved in the family's social activities. In particular, the husband and wife often share common activities. In closed families little sharing exists. There is always a distance. Dad does his "thing," mom does hers, and rarely do they share common social activities. In fact, they frequently protect their activities from intrusion by the other. Rarely do they share their experiences, whereas in open families, even if the members are not actually engaged in one another's activities, they enjoy talking to each other about their experiences.

Previous Crises

An adaptive response to life necessitates taking risks, inviting new challenges, and being open to accepting failure as a valuable learning experience. The open family provides greater exposure to the problems that can arise whenever anything new is attempted. Open families frequently have more collective exposure to crises than do closed families that attempt to avoid risks. The closed family's emphasis on stability prohibits the more flexible "let's try it" response, and thereby limits its experience in working through disappointments, frustrations, and temporary set backs, as well as more frightening changes. The open family is therefore more comfortable and experienced with change than the closed family.

Knowledge

Knowledge comes from experience, the seeking out and sharing of information with others. The adaptive family openly discusses possible crises before they occur. Substance abuse, violence, relationship issues, sexuality, or the birth of a new child are just some of the issues that adaptive families talk about in the hope of preventing a crisis, or at least being better prepared should one occur. Maladaptive families fear such discussions. "If you talk about it, it's going to happen," is a response reflective of a maladaptive family system. If there is a "discussion" in a maladaptive family it is usually one way, from adult to child, with no opportunity for the child to express his/her opinion. The communication is more of a directive—"You will do this or think this way"—with little thought given to the eliciting of the child's thoughts, feelings, or ideas.

Network

The adaptive family maintains a healthy interaction with extended family members and/or friends, and welcomes the support of others. Maladaptive families do not share their lives or experiences with others. They do not ask for help and have a difficult time accepting help when it is available.

Summary

The list below shows the potential responses of a maladaptive family to a crisis. The opposite of each of these responses would be an adaptive response. These include both the family system responses and family processes.

- Emotionally detached, cold, aloof
- Emotionally explosive, unpredictable, helpless, and/or hopeless
- Unwillingness to communicate
- Unwillingness to ask for help or accept help
- Closed to new ways of coping
- Absence of family involvement in decision making
- Inability to alter roles, responsibilities, or expectations during crisis
- Denial, withdrawal or avoidance of inherent conflicts within a crisis
- Loss of parental direction, guidance, support
- Scapegoating, blaming
- Use of substances

A number of attitudes can be extrapolated from these maladaptive responses. Those who use these responses believe the following.

- If we don't talk about it, it will go away.
- Talking about it only makes it worse.
- This is our business, not anyone else's.
- If we can't handle it ourselves, it can't be handled.
- The only one who needs to bother with this is the person with the problem.
- The best way to handle a conflict is to ignore it.
- The more emotional you get the worse the problem gets.
- I don't care what you do as long as it doesn't destroy our image in the neighborhood.
- If you don't do it my way, get out.

All families utilize these responses at times. In assessing the maladaptive level of a family, the greater the number of maladaptive functions present, the greater the risk of the deterioration of the family, and of the prolonging of the crisis into a chronic condition. This view of these family functions and processes will become the basis for both assessment and for determining appropriate intervention(s).

Finally, all families experience crises. They may anticipate some of them, but many crises can't be prevented. Families can minimize the risk that crises will become dangerous to members, and, if possible, can approach them as opportunities to learn, grow, and strengthen the family unit and each member in that unit. If a family cannot approach a crisis as an opportunity to learn, however, then little will be learned and an opportunity to strengthen the family will be lost.

REFERENCES

Caplan, G. (1964). *Principles of preventive psychiatry*. New York: Basic Books.

Hill, R. (1958, February–March). Genetic features of families under stress. *Social Casework, 39*(2–3), 139–150.

Pasewark, R. A., & Albers, D. A. (1972, March). Crisis theory in search of a program. *Social Work*, pp. 70–77.

Rapoport, L. (1962, June). The state of crisis: Some theoretical consideration. *Social Service Review, 36*(2), 212-213.

Rooney, J. L. (1958, February-March). Special stress on low-income families. *Social Casework, 39*(2-3), 150-158.

Steele, W. (in press). *Developing crisis response teams in schools.* Holmes, FL: Learning Publications.

4

Review of the Stages of Intervention

In this chapter we will review the twelve stages of intervention. To some degree all twelve stages must take place in the initial interview. This interview may be limited to an hour, or, depending upon the crisis being presented, continue beyond an hour. This will be discussed in Chapter 5. We will point out the goal of each stage, and then in subsequent chapters provide specific techniques and aids that can be used to achieve these goals so as to be able to move on to subsequent stages.

In our review it will appear as if the crisis worker can engage one stage at a time, complete the work on that stage, and then move to the next. In practice this may not be as orderly a process. The worker will move in and out of the different stages, depending upon a host of influences, but upon completion of the interview will have engaged each stage. Subsequent interviews may focus more on some stages than others. The stages identified here below have been extrapolated from a review of the literature concerning various crisis strategies, as well as from the authors' experiences in school settings.

1. Structuring the interview.
2. Defining the family's understanding of the crisis.
3. Defining the intervenor's understanding of the crisis.

4. Determining the nature of the family system.
5. Determining boundary inhibitors, subsystem inhibitors, process inhibitors, and strengths.
6. Assessing the level of danger.
7. Developing a different cognitive understanding (perception) of the crisis for the family.
8. Identification, acceptance, and management of the feelings precipitated by the crisis.
9. Engaging the family in the problem-solving process.
10. Determining and accepting the solutions to be engaged.
11. Setting time tables and rehearsing the chosen solution.
12. Soliciting feedback as to the status of the family at the conclusion of the session.

STAGE ONE: Structuring the Interview

Goals:
1. Minimize the increase in anxiety.
2. Minimize further family deterioration.
3. Establish the credibility of the worker.
4. Define the parameters of the crisis intervention process and the type of interaction expected between the intervenor and family.
5. Empower the family.
6. Reach a consensus as to the value of continuing the process.

The initial interview is critical to the outcome of the intervention process. If ground rules, roles, responsibilities, and expectations are not made clear, the possibility of a positive resolution is significantly reduced. Families in crisis should act as if they are making a major purchase. They should be clear about what they are purchasing, how it works, what guarantees, if any, exist, what they can do to prolong the life of their purchase, as well as on what their purchase cannot be expected to deliver.

Families in crises, therefore, need to know what the intervenor can deliver, how it will be delivered, what they as a family can do to help make the results more meaningful and longer lasting, what the intervenor cannot be expected to deliver, when they can expect to see results, and what they can do if the process simply is not working. If the family is clear on these issues they can make an informed commitment to the intervention process. Their level of anxiety may even be reduced, and their sense of control over the current crisis reinstated significantly enough to help prevent any further deterioration.

STAGE TWO: Defining the Family's Understanding of the Crisis

Goals: 1. Identify possible distortions of the realities of the threats the crisis is precipitating.
2. Identify possible distortions of the perceived causes of the crisis.

Perceptions do not necessarily reflect reality. Perceptions, however, do reflect the perceiver's own sense of what is real. It is this perception of reality that initiates a person's responses to a crisis situation. Determining these perceptions is critical to an assessment of the appropriateness of the responses being observed. In a crisis certain observations may seem to reflect inappropriate, or even marginal, behavior if the intervenor does not understand how that individual or family is perceiving their situation. Formulating an assessment on the appropriateness or inappropriateness of behavior without understanding the individual or family's perceptions can adversely affect the appropriateness of an intervenor's recommendations.

STAGE THREE: Defining the Intervenor's Understanding of the Crisis

Goals: 1. To identify those perceptions that may need changing to reflect the reality of the situation.

2. To identify the reasons as to why this crisis is occurring so as to target those areas that need corrective action if a healthy resolution is to be reached.

The intervenor's perception of the crisis may be in direct conflict with the family's perception. This must be understood so that the intervenor will be alert and able to respond to those areas that will need to be addressed in order to correct any misdirected responses. By identifying what the family understands to be the crisis the intervenor can assess which components of the crisis can be most easily resolved, strengthened, or referred for more intensive, longer term intervention. The intervenor's understanding of the crisis, coupled with his or her sense of the family's perception of it, will help the entire process to become more focused and to result in clearer, more realistic expectations of what can be accomplished.

STAGE FOUR: Determining the Nature of the Family System

Goal: To identify the specific nature of the family system.

Knowing whether a system is largely closed, open, or random will contribute to the intervenor's decisions regarding the choice of intervention strategies that are most likely to bring about a satisfactory resolution. When the intervenor knows that he/she is working with a closed system, for example, he/she will understand the importance of seeking the support of the major authority in that system, as well as the importance of stressing an orderly intervention process, rather than give all of the family members the opportunity to arrive at their own decisions as to what solutions are to be attempted. The first will elicit a more supportive response, the second a more defensive one.

STAGE FIVE: Determining Boundaries, Subsystems, and Process Inhibitors and/or Strengths

Goals: 1. To further identify those factors that will either become potential barriers to resolution or enhance the likelihood of a healthy resolution of the crisis.
2. To prioritize those areas needing the most immediate attention.

Stages two, three, four, and five become the bases for the initial assessment and subsequent intervention recommendations and/or strategies. They provide the information needed to determine the direction and style of the intervention to be provided and enable the intervenor, as much as is possible, to engage in those specific interventions designed to protect the family from further "at-risk" behavior and/or deterioration.

STAGE SIX: Assessing the Level of Danger

Goals: 1. To determine the potential for lethal and/or self-destructive behavior.
2. To ascertain the intervention needed to prevent lethal and/or self-destructive behavior.

With any crisis comes the potential for danger. This danger may be of a very lethal nature, such as suicide or homicide, or of a violent nature, such as physical abuse and/or assaultive behavior. While lethal danger may not be likely, any crisis, depending upon the extent of the family's vulnerability and hopelessness, creates the potential for such behavior and therefore this must always be addressed. When the potential for lethal and/or self-destructive behavior exists intervention must first address that potential and provide whatever safeguards are possible. The level of danger may not become apparent during the first five stages, but this assessment needs

to be completed before moving forward with any actual intervention strategies.

STAGE SEVEN: Presenting a Different Cognitive Understanding of the Crisis for the Family

Goals: 1. To normalize the responses to the crisis, thereby
            minimizing the anxiety related to the fear of los-
            ing all control.
         2. To provide those in crisis with an explanation that
            suggests that the crisis situation can be stabilized,
            resolved, or managed without further deterioration.

It is critical to those in crisis to understand that first, their
reactions are appropriate given their situation, and second, that
theirs are not unlike the reactions others have had in similar
situations. This allows them to know they are not abnormal
and that the intervenor perceives their reactions and situations
to be ones he/she has experience working with and resolving.
    Members of families in crisis will tend to believe that other
individuals within the family are the source of the problems,
rather than understand that the entire system has become
problematic. However, each knowingly or unknowingly contributes to the ongoing crisis, and each can contribute to its
resolution. By developing for the family a different cognitive
understanding of the crisis, the potential for scapegoating,
and/or the placing of the responsibility for change on
another family member can be avoided.

STAGE EIGHT: Identification, Management, and Acceptance of Feelings Precipitated by the Crisis

Goals: 1. To minimize destructive and/or self-defeating ex-
            pressions of feelings.
         2. To channel feelings into the energy and support
            necessary for resolution activities.

Crises can bring the worst out in people. Aggressiveness, passive aggressiveness, projection, displacement, denial, blaming, and guilt, can overtake rational, practical, reality-based responses. These emotional responses are very understandable. They are typical reactions in the face of a threat, and they must be identified, diffused, and accepted as normal reactions to fear, vulnerability, and a sense of powerlessness and hopelessness. Those expressions that support, encourage, nurture, and applaud efforts to resolve the crisis without damaging relationships, however, must be substituted for them.

STAGE NINE: Engaging the Family in the Problem-Solving Process

Goals: 1. To educate the family as to a problem-solving process that can be used regardless of the crisis being presented.
2. To develop problem-solving skills in each family member.
3. To instill a sense of empowerment in family members.

The two major interventions used for crisis resolution are education and problem-solving. Stage seven speaks to the education process. The problem-solving stage is critical not only to the resolution of the current crisis, but to the prevention of future, unavoidable crises as well. Done correctly it can help keep future crises from overwhelming the family, and thereby keep family members from losing control or becoming dysfunctional. Problem solving is also at the core of an individual's ability to feel empowered, regardless of the crises being experienced. When one feels empowered he or she becomes more confident, more secure, and more hopeful, all of which can help to prevent the development of self-defeating and/or self-destructive responses to crises.

STAGE TEN: Identifying and Selecting the Problem— Determining and Accepting the Solutions

Goals: 1. To reach a consensus as to the solutions to be engaged.
2. To establish ownership of the arrived at solutions.

When one is in crisis the solutions are often not obvious. Families must be assisted in identifying what might appear to be very obvious solutions to the intervenor. Most individuals, including professional counselors, have very sketchy crisis problem-solving skills. Families are no different. They need to be taught how to go about solving problems when their usual methods are ineffective. It is this process that can give family members a sense of ownership of those arrived at solutions. When the solutions are successful family members can develop a sense of confidence in their ability to resolve future crises. However, because a family is a system, the decision to engage in a specific problem-solving method must be reached by consensus. Not everyone may agree that a single solution is the best solution, but through consensus all members can agree that a solution is worth trying and supporting. Agreement as to the value of any solution, therefore, may differ. But, as long as there is a consensus, and the effort is supported by all, this effort itself becomes a healthy, learning, and adaptive response to the crisis, regardless of the particular outcome of that solution.

STAGE ELEVEN: Setting the Time Table and Rehearsing the Chosen Solution

Goals: 1. To prevent the negative aspects created by inactivity during a crisis.
2. To prevent the negative aspects of the absence of structure or order during a crisis.

We have now come full circle. When a family presents itself as being in crisis it is seeking immediate solutions or actions that can help the members to manage their crisis. They need structure and order to avoid the further anxiety that can be caused by a disorderly environment. Initially, the intervenor provides the order, the structure, and the actions necessary to bring the crisis under management. The family's ability to act in an orderly, systematic fashion during a crisis enhances the likelihood that they will regain control and at least return to their level of functioning prior to the crisis. In this regard they are now becoming intervenors.

STAGE TWELVE: Reassessing the Family Status

Goals: 1. To prevent the misunderstanding of expectations, roles, and responsibilities.
2. To minimize doubts and assess the overall change in status between the initial and final stages of the interview.

A last minute check is always beneficial for the intervenor as well as for the family. This is the time to clarify any items that might prohibit or interfere with positive resolution. It provides the family with an opportunity to address any issues that the now complete interview process has brought to the surface. It also provides the intervenor with the opportunity to conduct a final assessment prior to the family's leaving. In some situations, for example, families will calm down during the interview, but when the interview is about to end the anxiety may escalate. The intensity of the anxiety being experienced by the family may indicate to the intervenor the need to arrange an appointment for the following day, or a time to call later to respond to any concerns the family may have. This last stage, therefore, provides both the intervenor and the family with the opportunity to rethink their determined recommendations.

SUMMARY

We reiterate that this process may not be as orderly as it appears to be in this discussion. The techniques for completing each stage (to be discussed in subsequent chapters) will, however, provide an understanding of how the intervenor can move in and out of various stages until the goals of each stage are completed. It may also appear from this brief discussion that the entire process might be a lengthy one that could not be included in a single session. Again, as the techniques and tools are reviewed, it will be seen that all of the stages can be comfortably covered in one session, and that subsequent sessions will return to each stage, but will spend less time in some and more in others.

ADDITIONAL READING

Caplan, G. (1964). *Principles of preventive psychiatry*. New York: Basic Books.

Golan, N. (1969, July). When is a client in crisis? *Social Casework*, pp. 389–394.

Golan, N. (1978). *Treatment in crisis situations*. New York: Free Press.

Heiney, S. P. (1988). Assessing and intervening with dysfunctional families. *Oncology Nursing Forum, 15*(5), 585–590.

Kerns, E. (1970, June). Planned short treatment: A new service to adolescents. *Social Casework, 51*(6), 340–346.

Madanes, C. (1988). *Strategic family therapy*. San Francisco: Jossey-Bass.

Malan, D. H. (1976). *The frontier of brief psychotherapy*. New York: Plenum Medical.

Perlmutter, R. A., & Jones, J. E. (1985, Spring). Problem solving with families in psychiatric emergencies. *Psychiatric Quarterly, 57*(1), 23–31.

Rapoport, L. (1967, March). Crisis oriented short term casework. *Social Service Review, 41*(38), 38–41.

Rapoport, L. (1970). Crisis intervention as a mode of brief treatment. In W. Roberts & R. H. Nee (Eds.), *Theories of social casework* (pp. 267–311). Chicago: University of Chicago Press.

Rapoport, L. (1971, February). Short term crisis intervention: An approach to serving children and their families. *Child Welfare, 50*(2), 101-107.

Walker, B. A., & Mehr, M. (1983, Summer). Adolescent suicide—a family crisis: A model for effective intervention by family therapists. *Adolescence, 18*(70), 285-292.

II

STAGES OF INTERVENTION

5

Preparing for the Interview: Supportive Procedures and Crisis Worker Profiles

The first three chapters established the value of using the crisis intervention and family system models in the school setting. The effectiveness of such an intervention will depend largely upon the crisis worker's ability to integrate these two models into the intervention process. In this chapter we will review the procedures that must be in place in order to support this crisis intervention approach, and the attributes that make for an effective crisis intervention specialist.

POLICY AND PROCEDURES

The following procedures support the crisis intervention process. If they are not in place the effectiveness of the crisis intervention model will be seriously diminished. The procedures that need to be in place relate to:

1. Immediate availability
2. Temporary suspension of the crisis worker's daily responsibilities

3. Backup coverage and support
4. Restrictions on the duration of interviews
5. Frequency of sessions
6. Crisis worker preparation
7. Engaging community resources
8. Liability issues in potentially lethal situations

Immediate Availability

Keeping in mind that families are the most amenable to help when they are experiencing their most intense level of vulnerability (anxiety, fear, pain), it is critical for the school crisis worker or team to respond immediately upon the identification of a crisis. Asking a family to wait even one day before a meeting can take place puts the worker at a disadvantage because the family may simply grab on to someone else or to some other form of coping that promises to eliminate and/or reduce the anxiety, fear, and pain caused by the threat of the crisis. This places the responsibility on school administrators to establish both a policy and a procedure that allow the crisis worker or team the flexibility to delay other duties until after the initial meeting with the family. Schools that have developed crisis teams have also developed a "team approach" with this in mind. It allows for an immediate response, and in many cases reduces the duration of the crisis because there is little delay in taking the action neccessary to stabilize the situation. Delays in response usually lead to greater dysfunctional behavior.

Keep in mind that some of the answers and/or suggestions that you provide initially may turn out to be less than helpful because you have not had the time to obtain all of the information necessary to give the most effective response. What those in crisis remember and respect, however, is that they were taken seriously enough to be given immediate attention. This is what establishes you as a caring individual, one whom they will be more likely to turn to when compared to those who make them wait. Recalling one of your own personal experiences with a crisis will validate this principle for you. You appreciate those who do something immediately, not those who say "let's wait to see what happens."

Temporary Suspension of Crisis Worker's Daily Responsibilities

No one staff person can be expected to intervene in every crisis. There must be several people who can rotate this responsibility. A single staff person will quickly burnout, or reach a crisis state him/herself. This is another reason why many schools are developing crisis teams.

No matter who is responsible for intervening in crisis situations, a procedure or mechanism must be in place that allows the intervenor to leave his or her current duties and attend to the crisis. Crisis workers simply cannot be effective if they are worried about what they have left to do that day. Because of the emotional intensity of a crisis, the worker must be able to focus as much of his or her energy as is possible on that situation. It is not likely that every crisis is going to create a serious backlog of work, but the worker must know that should a situation demand a good deal of time, his or her work can either be completed by someone else or finished by the worker at a later date.

Backup Coverage and Support

The above procedure creates another procedural need. There must be backup staff available to cover the situation when a crisis worker must leave to attend to a crisis. The backup may be the same person who completes the daily routine that the crisis worker is now not able to attend to because of the crisis involvement. There is also another role backup staff need to assume. No one can assess with certainty what kinds of behaviors might escalate during intervention. If a family member's behavior, for example, does begin to escalate in a way that may become potentially dangerous or disruptive to the intervention efforts with the rest of the family, the backup can meet and intervene with that member privately.

In most cases, however, the access to backup colleagues is more consultive in nature. Even the most seasoned worker can experience anxieties that may cloud or distort certain issues.

Always, before making any final decisions about recommendations, it is advisable to discuss what has taken place with a backup colleague. The backup can usually be more objective, and in most cases can identify an area or two that the intervenor did not cover. This process therefore benefits the intervenor as well as the family.

The backup can also help to arrange for referrals if necessary, call other involved parties, and validate the intervenor's decisions as related to assessment and intervention strategies. Basically, no crisis worker should be left with the sole responsibility for assessment and decisions related to intervention strategies and/or recommendations. These need to be joint responsibilities. The team approach is dealt with at length by Steele, who focuses on the value of the team approach in enhancing the crisis worker's effectiveness in assessment, intervention, and prevention as well as on the school's liability in potentially lethal situations such as suicide (Steele, in press).

Duration of Interviews

We are all familiar with the 50-minute hour. In a crisis the 50-minute hour simply does not work. The amount of time it takes family members to feel more in control of their fear and more hopeful of a positive outcome will determine the length of the initial interview. An interview under the crisis model, therefore, may be only an hour or two, but could possibly consume an entire day. The amount of time will depend upon the immediate danger, the complexity of the situation, the need to gather information, the availability of external resources, such as other family members, friends, or professionals, and finally, the ability of the family to agree upon the most immediate problem-solving solutions, and to gain a renewed sense of their ability to manage and work through the crisis. The average length of an initial interview runs about 1½ hours, but the flexibility to meet until the immediate danger is stabilized is critical. Specific intervention strategies will be addressed later.

Frequency of Interviews

A crisis is limited to 4-6 weeks. Therefore, interventions will also be limited to this period of time. The greatest number of interviews usually occur within the first 2 weeks. Thereafter, the interviews are less frequent. The principle used to determine the frequency of interviews is quite simple. The family is to be seen as often as is necessary to stabilize and/or return the family to their accustomed level of functioning. This may occur after one interview, or several may be needed. Some families may need to be seen two, three, or even four times during the first week. This is contrary to the usual practice of once a week counseling, but no different a response than if there was a medical crisis. This is just as real a crisis, and a family is going to be willing to do what is necessary to rid themselves of it.

Crisis Worker Preparation

Crises are as anxiety producing for crisis workers as for family members because a worker simply has no idea whether a situation will escalate and/or deteriorate before stabilization can be achieved. The behavior of family members during a crisis can sometimes seem very bizarre or even pathological. This is understandable if it is remembered that a person in crisis, terrified by his or her own vulnerability and in a panic, may resort to somewhat drastic defenses.

As a crisis worker you must be able to feel some comfort about your own areas of vulnerability. Crises will bring them to the surface no matter how much experience you have or how skillful you may have become as a professional. In most of these situations you will likely be able to maintain control over your own anxieties while still helping the family in crisis. Occasionally, however, the anxiety that family members create for you may reduce your effectiveness. Crisis workers must be able to acknowledge when their own anxiety becomes such that it is counter productive to a successful intervention. This is another benefit of having a crisis team. If a situation, such as child abuse, sexual assault, or the violent death of a family member, becomes too emotionally overwhelming, another team member can step forward and help out. These personal reactions can, in fact, be helpful to the other team member as a reference point for what the family members are also experiencing. We are all human and being human we simply cannot handle all situations with equal effectiveness.

Should you know beforehand that the family crisis is one that you are not emotionally prepared to handle, find someone who can immediately. If in the middle of an intervention you feel as if you may be "in over your head," it is appropriate to acknowledge to the family that their situation is one that one of your colleagues has more experience handling. In this situation you would team up with that person until such time as the family is comfortable with and has confidence in your colleague. You will not lose respect as long as you model behavior that shows that even though you may not be able to provide the help they need, you are not helpless or powerless in bringing that help to them. This is what gives you credibility as someone who cares.

Engaging Community Resources

Many crisis situations demand that the crisis team and/or worker be able to engage those community resources that can best assist with the crisis being presented. If the family is in crisis over the death of one of its members, the worker needs to have access to those with expertise in, as well as resources pertinent to bereavement. Such community resources can be used as consultants, or to provide emergency evaluations, supply resource information for the family, provide training to crisis workers in specific areas of concern, or provide support to the family during those hours when schools are not operating so that the family has 24-hour access to help. Be sure to identify such community resources, and to keep a list of the contact persons and the services they provide. A smart crisis worker will maintain and nuture these resources because without them he or she will, without a doubt, at times feel stranded.

Liability Issues

Every administration and crisis worker must be cognizant of the liability issues related to potentially lethal situations such as suicide, homicide, sexual and physical abuse, and neglect. Steele (in press) addresses the duty to inform and refer in these situations. Every policy should clearly identify these legal responsibilities and procedures, and should very clearly spell out what must be done should suicide or homicide be threatened or sexual or physical abuse and/or neglect be suspected. Most school systems today are aware of the issues related to sexual and physical abuse. They also need to be aware of the legal ramifications related to suicide and homicide.

CRISIS WORKER ATTRIBUTES

There are two areas that counselors, social workers, psychologists, and other helpers find difficult to engage when they first begin doing crisis intervention. Most find it difficult to be assertive and "problem-solving oriented" (Steele, in press).

Assertiveness

When people fearing for their lives ask for help they fully expect a direct, active, assertive response from the helper. They do not expect to hear, "What do you think needs to be done?" Most helping professionals have been trained to be nurturing, supportive, empathetic, and reflective, but not assertive. Certainly these other attributes are essential, but if the crisis worker cannot be assertive he or she will lose credibility with those who need someone to step in and take charge immediately.

Assertiveness demands a certain level of confidence and comfort in one's own ability to make decisions with limited information and a limited time to act. Doing nothing in a crisis is encouraging danger, while making a decision and acting on that decision will quickly reveal its appropriateness or helpfulness. Many people are so afraid of making inappropriate decisions that they make none. They forget that with each decision comes new information, which in turn allows for additional adjustments and decisions, which ultimately may resolve the presenting problem.

Without directness and assertive intervention the family in crisis is simply going to experience more anxiety and frustration, and may begin to ignore or refuse any further intervention attempts. Anyone who has a sense of what they can do to eliminate the threat that they experience during a crisis will act. Families in crisis are coming for help because every idea that they have had to correct the situation has failed. As soon is as possible they need and deserve to be given the necessary direction to help stabilize the situation. They then can become involved in additional problem solving, and thereby prevent such a situation from reaching crisis proportions in the future.

Problem Solving

At the core of the problem-solving model is the belief that no matter what the situation you are not powerless. There are always choices available. Some choices may be ineffective, but there are other choices that will bring resolutions. They just take some finding. Also, the choices that do not work can teach us a great deal. They teach us what does not work. This may seem overly obvious or simple because very few people see success as the process of making a number of incorrect choices until the correct choices emerge. It is critical for the crisis worker to be not only a problem solver. He or she must engage the family in the problem-solving model to drive home the point that people are never helpless or powerless as long as they continue to make choices until they discover what works.

The reality in crisis intervention work is that decisions must be made. Many of these decisions may be ineffective in resolving the situation, however, and so only by continuing the problem-solving, decision-making process is the resolution for removing, avoiding, or managing the crisis found.

These then are the policies, procedures, and major attributes that must exist if the intervention process is going to have the best possible chance to successfully resolve the presenting crisis. Certainly techniques and tools are also needed, but if those techniques and tools are not assertively utilized they become useless. The chapters to follow will introduce specific strategies, techniques, and tools that can be helpful throughout the stages of intervention. Again, however, if the assigned crisis worker cannot take an assertive role and engage the family in the problem-solving process, he or she will simply not be successful.

REFERENCE

Steele, W. (in press). *Developing crisis response teams in schools.* Holmes, FL: Learning Publications.

ADDITIONAL READING

Caplan, G. (1964). *Principles of preventive psychiatry.* New York: Basic Books.

Golan, N. (1969, July). When is a client in crisis? *Social Casework,* pp. 389–394.

Golan, N. (1978). *Treatment in crisis situations.* New York: Free Press.

Heiney, S. P. (1988). Assessing and intervening with dysfunctional families. *Oncology Nursing Forum, 15*(5), 585–590.

Kerns, E. (1970, June). Planned short treatment: A new service to adolescents. *Social Casework, 51*(6), 340–346.

Madanes, C. (1988). *Strategic family therapy.* San Francisco: Jossey-Bass.

Malan, D. H. (1976). *The frontier of brief psychotherapy.* New York: Plenum Medical.

Perlmutter, R. A., & Jones, J. E. (1985, Spring). Problem solving with families in psychiatric emergencies. *Psychiatric Quarterly, 57*(1), 23–31.

Rapoport, L. (1967, March). Crisis oriented short term casework. *Social Service Review, 41*(38), 38–41.

Rapoport, L. (1970). Crisis intervention as a mode of brief treatment. In W. Roberts & R. H. Nee (Eds.), *Theories of social casework* (pp. 267-311). Chicago: University of Chicago Press.

Rapoport, L. (1971, February). Short term crisis intervention: An approach to serving children and their families. *Child Welfare, 50*(2), 101-107.

Walker, B. A., & Mehr, M. (1983, Summer). Adolescent suicide—a family crisis: A model for effective intervention by family therapists. *Adolescence, 18*(70), 285-292.

6

Intervention Stages
One, Two, and Three

STAGE ONE: Structuring the Interview

When we are fearful of some perceived or real threat, what do we want? When we feel as if we are losing control, what do we want? When we are so anxious we can't think straight, what do we want? When we are feeling overwhelmed, what do we want? What we want and desperately need is for someone to prepare us for what might happen next. At a more basic level, we do not want anymore surprises or anything new to have to deal with on top of everything else.

Imagine yourself to be in crisis, feeling confused, overwhelmed, and fearful of losing control. It has been suggested that you seek help. You have never had counseling before, but you agree to an appointment. That decision has now presented you with an entirely new set of unknowns that further intensify your anxiety. When you walk through that counselor's door and first sit down, what is going to be the most helpful, most comforting introduction that the counselor can provide? Will it be a brief greeting and then the question, "So tell me what brings you here?" No. This will not reduce your anxiety. Will it be his or her introducing you to how this interview is to be conducted, telling you what he or she can provide for you, what will be expected from you, how long it might take, asking you if you have any questions as to how it all works, or questions about him or herself, and finally, if, with all of this information, you would like to begin or reconsider? Yes. This will help reduce your anxiety.

In a crisis state what we need is structured information so that we can feel somewhat prepared for what we are about to do or for what is about to be done to us. (By structuring the intervention process you can not only reduce patients' anxiety but also establish yourself as a sensitive intervenor, who respects their right to know what they are about to "purchase" from you). It can return a level of control to them, remove many of the unknowns and myths that people generally have about counselors and therapists, and allow them to begin to focus on and even anticipate an early resolution. With their anxiety level reduced they can refocus the energies used to combat their fears into resolving their crisis.

Several structuring statements follow. As you review them you will notice that they are based on the crisis intervention and family systems principles and/or intervention strategies discussed in the previous chapters. This is where theory is transformed into actual application. We suggest that you become familiar with these structuring statements. Add to them if you wish, and/or use the list as a checklist to be sure that you have covered all of these issues before actually moving into a discussion of the family's problems.

It has been our experience that counselors and helping professionals in general find this process difficult to implement. This is partially due to training that tends to ignore or shy away from such a direct approach. It is also partially due to the helper's anxiety that discussing such issues before moving into the problem areas, given emotional state of the patients, is often too much for family members in crisis to manage. The fact is that this structuring helps them to better manage their emotions, and so we strongly encourage its practice as a valid intervention strategy.

Structuring Statements

• We are going to approach this as a crisis situation and as such you can expect to have some resolution in 4-6 weeks.

• There are two possible outcomes of this process. The situation may be resolved. If the situation cannot be changed, you will have regained control so that the situation is no longer the threat to you it is now. The other possibility is that we will be unable to resolve this crisis. However, we will be better able to identify what is actually causing it and what is needed to resolve it. So we can, if necessary, bring in or refer you to the appropriate resource so that it can be resolved in the shortest period possible.

• We will meet as often as is necessary during the next 4-6 weeks, and as quickly as possible should you request an unscheduled visit. Difficulties are much easier to resolve when they arise, as opposed to having them go on for several days before getting to them.

• Some sessions may last longer than others. We will meet as long as is necessary to resolve the particular issue we are dealing with.

• Initially I will have many questions to ask all of you. The more information you can provide the easier it becomes for us to arrive at a solution.

• You may also ask me questions, and if you do I will be as direct as I can be and give you my honest opinions.

• If I do not have the answers to your questions I will tell you, and then find the answers by the next session, or while you wait if it is an urgent situation.

• You need to understand how I approach a family in crisis. Rarely does any one family member have the sole burden of the problem. A family is like any other organization, team, or group of people who work together. If one of the members is not fulfilling his or her role, living up to expectations and obligations, or failing to perform his or her duties, the entire organization, team, group, or family is put in crisis. Whenever one member of a family changes, or a person's condition changes, the entire family faces new challenges, changes, and choices.

• We will therefore work on not blaming any one person in this family for what is occurring, and look both at the problem that this crisis has created for each of you and at the ways that you as a family can pool your resources, learn from this crisis, and get back on track.

• I will not ask you to try any solution without first looking at what the possible consequences might be. If you are uncomfortable with the proposed solution we will simply work together to find another.

• Let me give you a warning. Some of our solutions may sound very good here in the office but fail miserably when you try to implement them. This does not mean that either you or I have failed, but only that the solution simply was not the best solution at this time. In that situation we just move to our next alternative.

• Sometimes in this process the crisis seems to get worse not better. This happens because as we begin to take a look at an issue other problems begin to emerge. This is also the time when families tend to give up. Keep in mind that when additional problems begin to emerge it means that we are making progress and clarifying how this crisis has effected each and every one of you. When we know this it is much easier to make decisions as to how best to resolve the crisis. So when things seem to be getting worse, let me know, but also remember that it is a sign of progress. Also, keep in mind that by the end of the 4-6 week period you will know much more about your situation, including what works, what doesn't work, and what you will need to do to maintain any progress we have made.

• Should a serious crisis arise and you feel you need assistance outside of our school hours I want to give you several numbers that you can call to get immediate assistance. I encourage you to call should this happen, and to call me the next morning so that we can be sure to resolve the situation.

• Before we conclude our session today I'm going to introduce you to some of my colleagues (team members). This is for your benefit. If for some reason I am not available when you need to meet with me, one of my colleagues will be able to help out. I will keep them apprised of our sessions so that they can be of help to me as well as to you should you need immediate attention. No one else will know of your situation. All information will be kept confidential and not be placed in your son's/daughter's public file.

• Also, before we conclude today you will know exactly what will be taking place during the next few days. This we will agree on together.

• I want you to feel free to let me know when you think I am way off base. I'm sure I may say some things that are, but if you do *not* let me know I will proceed on the basis that I am correct. This will not be helpful for either of us.

• Finally, there are some ground rules for our sessions. Because we are dealing with a crisis and you have fears about the worst that can happen, some of our sessions may become very emotional. I must have your agreement on the following conditions:

1. There will be no physical contact, like hitting, shoving, or punching.
2. Initially yelling may be unavoidable, but when I ask everyone to stop I expect you to so that we can all collect our thoughts.
3. Should you want to discontinue counseling I ask that you let me know here in my office so that I can provide you with a summary of my thoughts as to what might be helpful for you in the future.
4. Finally, I want you to know that should you feel like discontinuing counseling because you simply are not satisfied or feel that we do not understand one another, tell me this. I will not take offense, and I will give you several referrals. Counseling is no different from seeking the services of a physician. If you don't like or trust a physician, you find one that you can trust.

• I know that I have given you a lot to think about, but I want you to know how this process works, what you can expect from me, and what I expect from you. Are there any questions? If not, how about we start by one of you telling me more about what has been happening.

This kind of structuring may seem like more than enough, but family members appreciate and respect it. Rarely are those in crisis told what is about to happen by intervenors, whether they be counselors or physicians. Nor are clients usually "empowered" by counselors as to their participation in the counseling process, or communicated to with such directness about the expected length of counseling, the possible outcomes, their role as it relates to interactions with the intervenor, or the reassurance available should the process not work as planned. In this case the intervenor will assist the family to find someone else who may be more helpful, rather than challenge the family's judgement. For these reasons we strongly encourage the use of this structuring process.

STAGE TWO: Defining the Family's Understanding of the Crisis

Defining the Crisis

Who determines what constitutes a crisis—the family, the school, or both? From a clinical view point, if people present themselves as facing a crisis they are in crisis, despite an intervenor's objective assessment to the contrary. A teenager may present as being in crisis because of the break up of a "long-term" relationship with a boy- or girlfriend. Objectively, the adult counselor sees this not as a crisis, but rather as a temporary, situational problem with no serious dangers because there will be many more boy- or girlfriends to come. The teenager, however, perceiving this loss to be serious and permanent, may in his or her crisis entertain very self-defeating or even self-destructive thoughts and/or behaviors such as suicide. From this view point, it is the individual and/or family that defines what constitutes a crisis.

A school may decide to define for itself what constitutes a crisis, such as a multitude of serious presenting problems, or a shortage of staff, and/or a lack of expertise in a specific area. They may decide that divorce, or running away, or a decline in a student's grades does not constitute a family crisis, whereas suicide, violence, sexual abuse, or sudden death does. A school may develop a priority response list and base their responses on a triage model so that certain situations result in an immediate response, while others are put on a waiting list. Each school will need to find a way to define what constitutes a crisis because every crisis demands an immediate response on the part of the crisis worker and/or team. Some schools may allow the family to define a crisis and then respond to whatever situation presents itself. Defining what constitutes a crisis, therefore, is an individual process for each school. Perhaps the only guideline for schools struggling to define when they will respond is that they must respond to any situation that has the potential for a lethal outcome.

Once the school determines a family's situation to be a crisis, and the meeting has been set and the structuring completed, the crisis worker must begin by determining the family's understanding of its situation. There are a series of questions that can help to reveal the family's understanding of the crisis, its causes, its dangers, its potential victims, the changes needed, and the possible resources that may be needed to resolve the crisis.

Questions for Defining Family's Understanding of Their Crisis

Following each question is a brief explanation of what each question is designed to reveal.

1. *We were not aware that any problems existed before today. Perhaps there were problems, but we did not recognize them, so what brought you here today as opposed to a week ago?*

Comment: The ability of the family to ascertain the original event that threw them into crisis, their possible minimization of the seriousness of events, the degree to which subsequent anxiety has distanced them from the primary cause and caused secondary issues to become the focus, and the degree of openness or defensiveness related to the confronting of the pain and fear that accompany the loss of control that this crisis has precipitated.

2. Do you have any ideas about what started this?
Comment: The ability of the family to partialize or focus on an agreed upon cause, and the degree to which family members differ in their understanding of the problem.

3. What were your initial reactions and what are your reactions, thoughts, and concerns now?
Comment: The extent of the family's coping skills and its self-defeating or destructive nature, if present.

4. Why do you think that this crisis is not going away?
Comment: The ability to assess what is needed or the degree to which they are feeling totally overwhelmed and in need of immediate answers. It also provides further insight into their ability to problem solve.

5. What have you tried to do?
Comment: More on the level of or availability of appropriate/inappropriate coping skills.

6. How does it leave you feeling?
Comment: The ability to identify, accept, and talk about feelings.

7. What does it make you feel like doing?
Comment: The potential for self-defeating or self-destructive behavior if the situation cannot be resolved. It also reveals the level of desperation and the degree of insight into the range of choices still available to them.

8. Is there anyone else involved—relatives, friends?
Comment: Assesses the level or extent of support as well as

the openness of the system to seek help from any available supports.

9. *What makes this situation more difficult than others that you have faced?*

Comment: Reveals again the level of desperation, as well as those areas that they have never before dealt with, and the level of distortion concerning the seriousness of these new problems.

10. *Do you think that this is an uncommon situation for families? Do you feel that you have handled it like most families would? (explain)*

Comment: The degree to which they perceive themselves to be approaching abnormal behavior, and the distorted perceptions they may have related to their reactions as being normal or abnormal given their situation.

11. *Who or what is hurting you the most right now?*

Comment: Identification of those persons or conditions that may need immediate attention and/or may be being used as "scapegoats," the degree of pain being experienced, and the anger, desire to hurt back, or fear being generated by others or specific conditions.

As is evident by the questions, assessment is already beginning. Some of these answers can be used to determine the levels of risk. Each question is designed, however, to provide a fairly comprehensive picture of family members' unique responses to this situation based upon their perceptions, their reactions, and their understanding of what is happening. Most often their perceptions will somewhat distort the dangers, the degree of seriousness, the degree of abnormality of their own reactions, and the cause of the crisis.

There may be additional questions that might arise as a result of the answers the family provides. What these questions will provide is the information you need when you enter stage seven and attempt to help the family understand their situation more appropriately.

STAGE THREE: Defining the Intervenor's Understanding of the Crisis

As a result of stage two you are already beginning to formulate your own ideas as to what is actually taking place, as well as what needs to take place, for resolution to occur.

Defending Against the Real Problem—Loss

The presentation by the family will frequently be a defense against what is actually taking place, which is often a reaction to a significant loss. Suicide, for example, is a life threatening crisis, but it may mask a deep reaction to a loss of hope. The loss of hope is the real crisis. Protection must certainly be given to prevent suicidal behavior, but if the real crisis—the loss of hope—is not addressed and replaced with some hope, as minimal as it may be, a suicide attempt is likely.

Family violence may be the presenting crisis, but again the underlying "real" crisis is an individual or family's fear of losing all control. Violence may seem to be the only choice available to overcome that fear of control being lost. Loss comes in many forms, and most people defend against the pain and fear that accompany any significant loss.

Table 6.1 lists the symptoms that can emerge following a loss. They often become the presenting problem, but are caused by the significant loss. The family's acceptance that the crisis they are experiencing is a result of a loss often becomes the focus of the intervention. The loss could be one they have experienced but have left unresolved, minimized, or altogether avoided because of the overwhelming pain and fear that any such loss can create.

The entire focus of crisis intervention is to help the family to identify the loss to realize that this loss has actually precipitated what they are now experiencing in their crisis, and to educate them as to the common reactions to loss. Then problem-solving concerning both the immediate crisis situation and the emotional pain and fear initially created by their loss can begin to occur. Steele (in press) devotes an entire book to

TABLE 6.1. Symptoms Following a Loss

1. Fear of personal survival
2. Separation anxiety
3. Impaired ability to make emotional attachments
4. Sadness
5. Anger
6. Guilt/shame/despair
7. Problems with control issues
8. Drop in developmental energy
9. Loss of self-esteem
10. Feelings of futility
11. Inability to concentrate
12. Hyperactivity
13. Sleep disturbance
14. Enuresis in children
15. Depression
16. Daydreaming
17. Withdrawal from peers
18. Repeated somatic complaints
19. Self-injurious behavior
20. Suicidal tendencies
21. Death fantasies
22. Traumatic dreams
23. Lessened interest in play or other usually enjoyable activities
24. Feeling more distant from parents or friends
25. Not wishing to be aware of their feelings
26. Increase in anxious attachment behavior
27. Startle reactions (sounds, smells, related to incident)
28. Avoidance behavior
29. Confusion and fear of one's own thoughts or reactions
30. Illusionary experiences of the deceased
31. General mistrust of others
32. Fear of ever allowing a close relationship
33. Prolonged anger, rage, hate, revenge, bitterness, resentment

Note. These symptoms are seen in both children and adults. Items 1–11 are from Jewett (1982), 12–14 from Zeanah and Burk (1984), 15–21 from Trent (1985), 22–30 from Pynoos and Nader (1988), and 31–33 from Kubler-Ross (1985).

trauma and loss, and discusses what helpers need to know to help families and children cope appropriately with loss.

The following are questions designed to help the intervenor identify the precipitating loss and subsequently reach an understanding of the actual crisis facing the family. Following each question is a brief explanation of what the question is designed to reveal.

1. What unexpected, unwanted, unfamiliar, or new situation or condition has occurred in the past two weeks?

Comment: Generally, by the time an unresolved crisis has manifested itself to the point where people ask directly for help or are observed to be needing some assistance, two weeks have passed since the actual event occurred. By specifically defining an event as "new," "unfamiliar," "unwanted," or "unexpected," the counselor can help the family members to recall loss situations that they would not otherwise have identified as the cause of what they are now experiencing.

2. Has anything new, unfamiliar, unwanted, or unexpected happened to anyone else you know?

Comment: On some occasions events do not happen directly to the person or family in crisis, but rather to someone they know, yet an individual might react as if he or she was the actual victim. The suicide death of a friend, a violent death, or a sudden, accidental death, for example, can trigger a crisis in a surviving friend or family. This question addresses the possibility that the crisis being presented was triggered not by something occurring within the family, but instead by events outside of the family.

3. Have you ever felt like this before? If so when, and what was happening?

Comment: The current crisis may have its roots in a previously unresolved loss, the effects of which are now being triggered by another event that compounds the initial loss with a more recent loss. A family may be in crisis because their teenage daughter is pregnant. Upon further investigation, however, it is revealed that either the mother was pregnant as a teen and/or the father impregnated another woman, and that neither of those events was satisfactorily resolved. These unresolved issues spill into and further intensify the current crisis.

4. *What other problems has this created for you?*
Comment: This question may address significant areas of vulnerability that have emerged as the result of the crisis, so that more than one issue of loss is currently being confronted. A father, for example, is laid off and has been unable to find work. As a result of his unemployment his spouse develops feelings of resentment that prevent her from providing the necessary support. The husband now must contend with the additional loss of support from his spouse, and the children in the family must contend with the loss of the security and/ or comfort that was still available to them in the early stages of the unemployment period.

5. *Have there been any changes because of this situation?*
Comment: In this question you may need to suggest specific areas of change, as the anxiety present during a crisis may blind or block those in crisis from remembering changes that have taken place. This question can help them to better focus their attention on specific areas. Changes could occur financially, socially, physically, spiritually, occupationally, academically, in personal relationships, or in other family relationships. Remember, what may not seem like an appropriate cause for a crisis to you as an intervenor may be a significant cause for those in crisis, and vice versa.

6. *What positive changes have occurred in the past several weeks?*
Comment: This question may or may not need to be asked. The answers usually reveal (if nothing else) helpful information related to assessing the family's strengths. Neither individuals nor families usually attribute a crisis to anything positive. As we discussed in previous chapters, however, any change, including a positive change, presents new challenges and choices and may create a crisis if an individual or family is at a loss as to how to respond and/or adjust to that positive change.

An adolescent male, for example, is a natural at football. By his senior year he has won numerous awards and is being offered scholarships by colleges. During that period, however, his behavior and personality change (loss), leaving parents unsure as to how to respond (loss). Prior to graduating he is picked up by the police for drinking in the back seat of a car. Neither he nor his parents realized the pressures he had been under. As a result of this positive change he faced new pressures from friends, felt he was being pushed into a leadership role, and had to deal with a new set of expectations. He was not prepared to cope with these rapid changes. In this situation the drinking is presented as the most immediate crisis, but its root cause is the loss he experienced when he was catapulted into "fame," if you will, and faced new challenges, choices, and changes that he was not equipped to handle (loss).

Again, there may be additional questions that emerge as a result of the answers that these questions bring out. The answers to questions in both stages two and three should provide the information you need to formulate the direction you will be taking, and asking the family to take, when you reach the problem-solving stages. They will also identify for you those areas that will need to be addressed in stage seven when you ask the family members to look at their situation differently.

REFERENCES

Jewett, C. L. (1982). *Helping children cope with separation and loss*. Boston, MA: Harvard Common Press.

Kubler-Ross, E. (1985). *On children and death*. New York: Collier.

Pynoos, R. S., & Nader, K. (1988). Psychological first aid and treatment approach to children exposed to community violence: Research implications. *Journal of Traumatic Stress, 2*(4), 445–472.

Steele, W. (in press). *Developing crisis response teams in schools*. Holmes, FL: Learning Publications.

Trent, B. (1985, December). Helping children cope with death. *Canadian Medical Association Journal, 133,* 1157–1161.
Zeanah, C. H., & Burk, G. S. (1984, January). A young child who witnessed her mother's murder: Therapeutic and legal considerations. *American Journal of Psychotherapy, 37*(1), 132–145.

7

Intervention Stages
Four, Five, and Six

At this point in time you may already have enough information collected to determine the nature of the family system, the boundary, the subsystem, process inhibitors and/or strengths, and the level of danger present. The process demanded of the family while moving through the first three stages may itself help to formulate an assessment without further questioning.

Stages four through six may be very brief in duration because of the information that the preceding stages have revealed. On the other hand, depending upon the level of danger present and the family's potential for self-destructive and injurious behavior, a more extensive and focused assessment may be necessary. The level of danger may in fact be such that an immediate referral to an outside clinical setting, one able to provide emergency measures if necessary, is the only remaining course left for the school. If this is the situation, then stages four through twelve will become significantly abbreviated.

If not, stages four, five, and six are critical to the entire intervention process. Without an assessment the information obtained cannot be validated. This will leave the intervenor on shaky ground regarding the appropriate utilization of the information, and will make it difficult to ensure the safety and well-being of the family members. Also, without an assessment the intervenor is vulnerable to a maze of liability issues.

NOT A CLINICAL SETTING

A school is not a clinical setting. Nor is it given the responsibility or the authority to determine the clinical assessment and treatment of families in need of counseling. It is a setting, however, that is responsible for recognizing and identifying situations that are potentially dangerous to its students, for providing a brief examination to verify the potential presence of such danger, and for providing the appropriate warning and referral if a danger appears life threatening. As long as any potential life threatening issues have been addressed and referred for further assessment, the school is authorized, if you will, to provide guidance and support via the process of educating those in crisis about the information available that has helped others in similar situations (i.e., parenting skills, problem-solving skills). The school, in fact, can play a major educative and supportive role, supplementing and reinforcing any outside treatment that is being provided.

The assessment stages, therefore, are designed primarily to identify the presence of potentially life threatening behaviors that demand further outside clinical assessment, and secondarily, to identify those aspects of the family's systematic way of processing a crisis that need addressing if the crisis is to be resolved.

THE SCHOOL ASSESSMENT

The school assessment is designed to reveal the presence of imminent danger, or, if there is doubt about the presence of such danger, to evaluate the need to refer an individual or family for further assessment. In the absence of imminent danger it is designed to identify those areas that can be addressed and aided via the education and problem-solving process within a 4- to 6-week period of time. These are the issues that will be addressed in this chapter.

STAGE FOUR: Determining the Nature of the Family System

As indicated earlier, you may have already determined by the family's responses to questions during the earlier stages whether they operate as a closed, open, or random system. If you have not made this assessment, or need further verification, return to Table 2.1, "Family System Characteristics," found in Chapter 2 and also available in the Appendix. A brief review of this chart may be sufficient to substantiate your assessment. Keep in mind, however, that this is a guide. There may be some areas that are closed, while others are open or random. What you're assessing is the overall pattern of responses. Do their responses, in other words, constitute mostly closed, open, or random responses? Although there will be systems that are clearly closed, open, or random, usually there will also be some cross over of responses.

The following are a series of questions that can be asked in each of the ten areas listed. These may elicit the information necessary to further identify and/or validate the type of system response engaged in each area.

1. **Rule:** How and who makes the rules in your home?

   The response will indicate the type of system.
   Closed response: Authoritarian in nature.
   Open response: Negotiable in nature.
   Random response: Permissive in nature.

2. **Focus:** How do you want others to see your family?

   Closed response: No matter what difficulties we may be having we want others to see us as being together and strong.

Open response: We want to be seen as a happy family,
                      but of more importance to us is how
                      each of us is doing.

Random response: It doesn't matter to us. We all have
                      our own individual pursuits. We
                      probably aren't like families that
                      spend a lot of time together.

3. **Affection:** In what ways do you usually express affection?

   The response will indicate the type of system (see
   Table 2.1).

4. **Goal:** What is the major goal your family strives to
   achieve and maintain?

   Closed response: Stability, security.

   Open response: We're flexible. Our goals change.
                       We're concerned about stability and
                       security, but the individual goals of
                       each member are probably more im-
                       portant.

   Random response: We try to pursue new experiences and
                       adventures.

5. **Ambiguity:** Do you like change?

   Closed response: We handle it. Change is okay, but we
                       don't like surprises.

   Open response: You can't avoid change. Everything
                       changes, so we work with it and make
                       the best of it.

   Random response: Changes are exciting. You've got to
                       take risks. If you're afraid of change
                       you're afraid of life.

6. **Conflict:** How do you manage conflict?

   The response to this question will reflect the characteristics
   identified in "Rule," "Ambiguity," "Decison making,"
   "Information processing," and "In a Crisis" in Table 2.1.

7. **Decision making:** When there is a major decision to be made how is it made and who makes it?

   The response will indicate the type of system (see Table 2.1).

8. **Information process:** How does information usually get passed on in your family?

   The response will reflect the response in "Rule," "Decision making," and "Communication" in Table 2.1.

9. **Communication:** Would you say that everybody knows everyone else's business in your family, or do you tend to believe that not everyone needs to know or should know everyone's business?

   Closed families may deny patterns of secretiveness, whereas open families will support openness and random families will support both secretiveness and openness. Patterns that emerge in "Rule," "Focus," "Affection," "Conflict," "Decision making," and "Information processing" will likely align themselves with the communication pattern characteristic of each system. This is a question, therefore, that may not need to be asked because its probable answer will be observed throughout the intervention process and "fit" with the overall systems pattern of response in these other areas.

10. **In a crisis:** The previous nine questions will reveal the patterns reflected in each of the system descriptions in this category (see Table 2.1).

Summary

It is important to define, if possible, the system responses most frequently used so as to determine the approach to be used in the intervention process, as well as to identify those areas that may need to be avoided, encouraged, or mirrored throughout the intervention process. For instance, the closed family system will obviously present the greatest resistance to change. The goal with them will likely be to return the family to its former level of functioning without challenging those areas that would lead to the emergence of more resistance.

Remember that time is short and that you are not providing long term or clinical intervention. You are going to try to align solutions to the style that the family most often uses when faced with change, so as not to intensify their anxiety by insisting on behavior that they seldom engage in. When working with a closed system, for example, you may become the decision maker and utilize your authority to outline any corrective measures, as opposed to encouraging all of the family members to participate in a resolution-finding, decision-making process. Keep in mind that your primary goal is stabilizating, not restructuring the family system. Knowing the type of system generally in use will help to sensitize you to approaches and processes to avoid. Closed families will want answers, while open families will want to process the possible answers and reach their choices by consensus. Random families will be as varied as the individuals within the system. Some will simply want to be told what will work, while others will want to explore and test the possibilities.

STAGE FIVE: Determining Boundaries, Subsystems, and Process Inhibitors and/or Strengths

Boundaries

Again, the inhibitors and strengths may have already been revealed by this time. If you are unsure of the potential inhibitors or strengths, the following questions can help to identify them.

1. How do you feel about getting help?
2. How do you feel about sharing your difficulties with an outsider?

3. How do you feel about paying for this service?
4. Do you believe talking really helps?

If we have adequately explained the differences between the systems, you will know that closed systems will respond negatively to these questions. They will not be comfortable asking for help, bringing in an outsider, or sharing their difficulties with extended family members. They will begrudge paying for such services. The open system will respond in just the opposite fashion, and the random family will probably be as rigid as the closed family in some of their beliefs and as flexible or participatory in other beliefs as the open family. Knowing the presenting boundaries will help you to know what boundaries are being placed on you as far as your choices concerning how to engage the family in the intervention process.

Subsystems

To assess the nature of the existing subsystems we refer you to the Chapter 2 discussion of subsystems and the exercise proposed using Figure 2.2. The Appendix includes this exercise and the tool needed under the stage five section.

Of primary importance is the determination of which patterns existed prior to the crisis and which developed during the crisis. A solid line may have connected father and son prior to the crisis (reflecting a solid relationship), but now this relationship is represented by a broken line (reflecting a tenuous relationship). Obviously the focus would be to reestablish the earlier relationship, or if this does not seem feasible, to strengthen the son's relationships with other individuals in the family who can provide what the father once provided.

Identifying changes in the subsystems also helps to identify both the losses the crisis precipitated and the losses that precipitated the crisis. As discussed earlier, the major thrust of the crisis model is to help individuals manage their reactions to the losses they have experienced. Once again you are looking for patterns. The patterns that exist in a subsystem will frequently reflect the overall family system. An open system will tend to have many solid lines interconnecting the majority of family members. Closed systems may have fewer solid connections and/or fewer multiple solid interconnections among members. The random system may reflect either the closed or the open system, depending upon the nature of the crisis, the individual's involvement in the crisis, and the issues it precipitates.

Processes

Specific processes have already been identified in stage four. (We also refer you to Chapter 2 and the segment on family processes that defines the positive elements of each of these processes.) In the limited time available to you to work with the family you want to "exploit" the positive processes already in place. Then, if the system can tolerate change, attempt to fix the processes that are broken. If it cannot, then you must rely on the processes that the family is the most comfortable using.

We also refer you to Chapter 2's discussion of the goals of the various systems. This discussion incorporates the key elements of each process area. The Appendix (section stage five) includes a subject rating chart that identifies the strongest and weakest processes of the family.

STAGE SIX: Assessing the Level of Danger

At this point you ought to have a good feel for the "real" crisis being presented, the distorted perceptions that the family has related based on their understanding of the crisis, the type of system you are encountering, the elements of the system you will utilize to problem solve, and the family processes you will engage. You may also have a sense of the level of danger that this crisis has precipitated, especially in relation to the potential for life threatening behavior. As discussed earlier, any question as to the presence of life threatening behavior automatically necessitates a referral to a clinical setting (i.e., community mental health, psychiatric emergency facility, or the children and adults services of your Department of Social Services). This is your legal duty, and will be further discussed in stages nine through twelve. Stage six of the Appendix provides information related to potentially violent and suicidal behavior. This work cannot possibly provide the variety of tools available for such problems as sexual or physical abuse, or psychotic destructive behaviors.

The following discussion on assessing the level of danger is taken from Steele (in press). "Family" can be substituted for the term "youth."

Assessing the Seriousness of the Crisis

Level 1. In assessing the seriousness of a crisis our first concern is for the safety of the youth in crisis. In other words, does this crisis put the youth in immediate danger? Is it causing the youth to engage in such overt self-destructive behavior as threatening suicide or violence, or in more covert but just as dangerous activities such as driving while intoxicated or provoking violent situations?

Level 2. The next level of concern would be related to behavior that does not place the youth in immediate danger but could have as lethal an outcome over a long term period, such as unsafe sex, weekend drinking at parties, occasional drug usage, or engaging in fighting.

Level 3. The third level of concern is related to those behaviors that may not lead to self-destructive outcomes but are self-defeating and in time could lead to self-destructive tendencies, such as a decline in school performance, social isolation, or repetitive lying, cheating, or stealing.

Additional Risk Factors. An additional area that affects the seriousness of the crisis is the availability or unavailability of support and resources. A youth with a nonsupportive family and few friends should be considered to be in a serious situation. An inability to immediately access outside agency support can also increase the danger, not only for the youth but for the intervenor as well.

Probably one of the most difficult aspects of crisis intervention is the changing of the condition or situation causing the crisis. Families are probably the greatest source of crisis for young people, and can also be one of the most difficult groups to access and change. Pushers, or friends who sell or use drugs, represent another example of a group that is difficult to reach or change. A youth who wants to go to college but whose family is financially poor is also in a situation that is difficult to modify. This is why crisis intervention is more concerned with the individual's response to the crisis than with actually manipulating the environment or the sources of the crisis, although this approach is never ruled out.

Therefore, the seriousness of the situation is determined by (1) the immediate danger to the individual's life, (2) the degree of support available to the individual, (3) the resources available to effect necessary change, and (4) the youth's willingness to engage in problem-solving activities. This is a purely subjective assessment but one with some validity for determining the degree of the difficulties hindering a resolution.

Assessing the Individual in Crisis

What is the likelihood that a youth in crisis will be able to avoid a self-destructive response to his or her crisis? How capable are youngsters of holding on until a solution is found that resolves the situation? Just what is the best intervention for a youth—hospitalization, psychiatric intervention, in-school intervention? Is the youth capable of taking control of the situation or must control be provided by others? Is the youth in imminent danger? Can they not only accept help but act on the help given? These are a few of the questions that intervenors must ask themselves during the initial interview.

Immediate Danger

Of first concern is any immediate danger to self and to others. Does this youth, in other words, have the resources available to hurt himself or others during this crisis? No one can predict with certainty that a youth will not attempt suicide or will not lose control and assault someone. Nor can anyone predict with certainty that a youth will not turn to drugs, run away, drop out of school, or engage in other self-destructive behaviors given the right set of circumstances.

To assess the immediate danger one can observe the risk factors that identify the potential for danger. A youth threatening suicide, for example, will tend to be less of a risk to himself if suicide is only an idea. He will likely be at greater risk if he has developed a specific plan. A youth is less at risk of turning to drugs if he is doing well in school, has non-drug-using friends, and is able to communicate with his parents, than he would be if none of these conditions existed. During the interview process there may be a need to ask questions specific to the presenting problem, such as suicide. The assessment, however, must also attempt to evaluate how capable that youth is of maintaining control in spite of the seriousness of the presenting problem. Although there are no absolutes to defining imminent danger, there are several key factors that can be assessed regardless of the seriousness of the problem being presented. One of the most useful of these is the recent history of the young person in crisis. The following list can be used as a guide when dealing with a youth in this situation.

If there is a history of similar behavior, the risk factor is likely to be higher.

If there has been a history of help, but the youth perceived that help negatively, the risk is more serious.

If there is a history or series of losses preceding this particular crisis, the risk factor increases.

If there is a history of poor impulse control, the risk is greater.

If there is a chaotic family history, the risk increases.

If there is a family history of resistance to change, the risk factor increases.

If there is a history of depression in one of the parents and/or in a single parent, the risk factor is higher.

If there is a current drug or substance problem, the risk is greater.

If there is a history of academic difficulties, the risk factor increases.

If the youth is unable to express or communicate his or her feelings and thoughts, the risk becomes greater.

If there is an inability to entertain recommendations, or a "yes but" response to recommendations and explanations, the risk is compounded.

If there is a refusal to accept recommendations, the risk is serious.

If there is an inability to compliment oneself or identify one's strengths, the risk intensifies.

If there is an inability to perceive others as not only caring but helpful, the risk becomes significant.

If there is an inability to engage in the problem-solving process, the risk level rises.

Some of this information may not be available to you, but any one of these items by itself indicates a fairly serious risk factor. Keep in mind that during noncrisis times these risk factors, although serious, will have less immediate impact than they will when the youth is in crisis because of the vulnerability, panic, fear, and anxiety he or she is now experiencing.

Assessing risk is a judgment call best made in consultation with team members prior to determining any immediate interventions. Making an assessment in isolation is a risk in itself and is not in the best interest of the youth, the intervenor, or the school. However, the presence of any of the above factors indicates a need for some immediate intervention strategies. Before the initial interview has been concluded the need for emergency interventions must be determined and, if necessary, implementation begun.

SUMMARY

The information accumulated up to this point will provide you with what you need to move on to stage seven. By now you should know the direction your interventions need to take, the problem areas needing the family's focus, and the processes that can be utilized to reach a healthy crisis resolution. The following chapters will focus on how you present and utilize this information, as well as those specific processes or intervention strategies that have proven most helpful in crisis situations.

REFERENCE

Steele, W. (in press). *Developing crisis response teams in schools.* Holmes, FL: Learning Publications.

8

Intervention Stages
Seven and Eight

Developing a different cognitive understanding of the crisis for the family is a pivotal task. At this point the crisis either becomes a significant danger or a significant opportunity. The danger can stem from a family's inability to open themselves to the idea that other, less obvious conditions or events might possibly have caused their current crisis, or to accept the normalcy of their reactions to their situation. The more rigid a family's stand against changing their viewpoint the more danger they place themselves in because they limit the possible solutions available to them.

There are three major opportunities available to families in crisis at this point. First, if a family can entertain a different understanding of the primary source of its crisis, intervention can be focused and direct. Rather than spending a great deal of time trying to overcome the very normal defenses precipitated by the crisis, this different presentation by the intervenor, if accepted, can frequently bring immediate relief by reducing the intensity of the family's anxiety. Any reduction of anxiety is going to result in clearer, more rational thinking, less panic or reactive behavior, and a renewed sense of control of the situation.

The second opportunity afforded families in crisis is the ability to learn that there are many different ways to resolve any crisis situation. Families often believe that there is only one choice available to them. In the crisis state the perception that there is only one course available is, as you can imagine, very anxiety producing. What if it does not work? Is all lost? Is what they fear the most about to happen? When family members are educated about the many possibilities always available to us in a crisis, however, anxiety levels are reduced and a sense of control returned.

The third available opportunity hinges on the family's ability to entertain the many possible solutions that will be revealed during the final stages. Families that are rigid and cannot, for whatever reason, entertain a variety of different possible actions, limit the extent of the possible resolutions. They deny themselves the opportunity to discover a problem-solving process that can be used in future crises, as well as the opportunity to reestablish their confidence in their capability to manage whatever crises might arise.

It is at this stage that the family chooses to close themselves off or to move ahead and seize the opportunity to emerge from this crisis a smarter, more empowered, stronger, and higher functioning family. It is at this point that the intervenor's expertise and ability to be helpful are crucial.

STAGE SEVEN: Presenting a Different Cognitive Understanding of the Crisis for the Family

Normalizing the Situation

When remembering a personal crisis can you recall if anyone ever said to you, "Look, given the situation you're faced with your reactions are not only very understandable but quite normal"? If you were so advised then you know the value of such a response. It helped you to know that you were not really out of control or "going crazy," but actually reacting appropriately to a situation you probably had no experience with. This kind of response helps you to realize that others do understand without minimizing the intensity of your feelings and/or reactions. It implies a sense of hope and reinforces the idea that others have faced similar situations, with similar reactions, and resolved them.

The intervenor can follow this statement with a brief explanation about the anxiety that is created by any new, unfamiliar, or unwanted situation because of the new challenges, changes, and choices it forces us to deal with or anticipate. This allows the individual or family in crisis to focus on the fact that their anxiety is normal and appropriate, since no one, including people faced with apparently positive changes, is totally free from anxiety. Everyone has questions such as "Will this work out? How well will I do? Will I end up looking like a fool? Will I be able to make the best of the situation? Will it all suddenly disappear?" To be told further that the way they are feeling and reacting does not mean that there is something wrong with them helps to reduce their fear of losing control. They simply have never been taught the kind of coping skills that would have resolved this situation. This helps to change their focus from their being somehow inadequate or a failure to their simply not having the knowledge they need to correct the situation, as others before them have done when faced with a similar situation.

This process of normalizing the situation not only helps them to understand their situation differently. It also makes them more amenable to what you have to say and removes you as a threat. The threat that they probably entertained about you is that you somehow perceive them to be severely troubled, inept individuals who have little chance of leading or normal life. This is rarely overtly expressed, but it is very much a fear that individuals carry with them into the initial interview. Normalizing the situation for them allows them to begin to perceive you as being a credible, caring, and helpful individual.

Providing an Acceptable Explanation for the Cause of Their Reactions

When an explanation of any kind is provided for what is happening it temporarily gives those in crisis something concrete to grab on to, and thereby reinstates their sense of control over the situation. Survivors after a suicide can never adequately answer the question "Why?" Not being able to answer this question delays their bringing closure to their grief because there is no place for them to focus their emotions. When a homicide or a death by accident or illness occurs, emotions can be directed at the cause.

Providing some explanation, even if it is somewhat incomplete, helps those in crisis to focus their emotions and arrive at a resolution much sooner than if no explanation seems available. The most logical, reasonable, and likely explanation of why they are reacting and feeling the way they are is that they are responding to a loss. This loss, whether real or feared, could be the loss of security, safety, hope, love, self-worth, or control over their own destiny. Whatever the crisis, one or several fo these losses will be experienced or feared as an impending reality. With any loss or anticipated loss comes the fear of the unknown or the unthinkable, and related feelings of grief. Fear unleashes a deep sense of vulnerability, while grief unleashes unwanted pain and its accompanying feelings of anger, guilt, denial, and hopelessness. The feelings accompanied by one's sense of vulnerability include fear, anxiety, helplessness, and powerlessness. As depicted in Figure 8.1., fear and loss feed and intensify the threat being experienced.

Again, these are all very normal and largely unavoidable reactions to loss. When this explanation is accepted, families in crisis can begin redefining their understanding of what has happened to them and seeing themselves as responding appropriately for what they are experiencing. They can actually begin to partialize or focus on the real crisis they are reacting to, the condition that has caused them to feel threatened.

Example: Arriving at a Different Cognitive Understanding of a Crisis

A family presents as the crisis the undesirable behavior of their teenage son, which has resulted in a call from school. The teenager's behavior, which has grown increasingly more

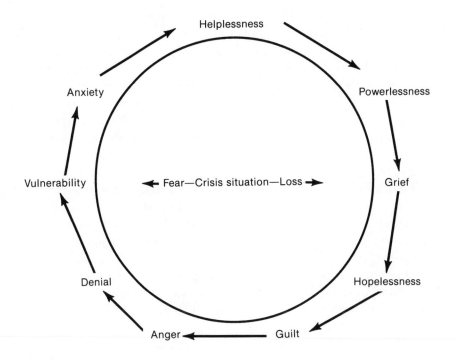

FIGURE 8.1. Circle of loss and fear.

unacceptable at school and at home, is the entire focus of the family's attention. They, of course, clearly indicate that if it weren't for their son's behavior the family would be doing fine.

Keeping in mind that the presenting problem is usually a defense against the underlying, precipitating cause of the crisis reaction, it is important to try to answer these questions: What has this youth lost that might be causing his behavior? What has the rest of the family lost as a result of this son's growing problem? In this example it is obvious that the parents experienced a loss of control over their son and constantly felt threatened by what might happen next. They were, therefore, feeling very appropriate vulnerability and intense anxiety over the loss of their ability to control their son. As a result of this loss, conflicts about how to best manage their son's behavior emerged between the parents, who were also experiencing a loss of control in their own relationship, as well as a loss of patience and control with the other children. This was appropriate, given that their normal coping skills failed to resolve the problem that developed into this crisis. The siblings also experienced a loss of comfort and security with their parents, who had become "different people" as a result of their reactions to their son's behaviors. These reactions were also appropriate given the changes they experienced in their parents, as well as from their brother. The family's responses were therefore normalized and defined as appropriate, given the fact that nothing they had tried had worked, and that despite their efforts their son's behavior was growing more destructive and was threatening the family's previous level of stability.

The son's behavior, although in need of correction, was not the major crisis. The major crisis was this family's "losses." The parents were feeling a loss of control, the siblings a loss of security, and the son was feeling such pressure to succeed and live up to his parents' expectations that he basically took control by going out of control—an appropriate reaction if he was feeling that too much was being expected of him. When this different cognitive perception of the crisis was presented to the family they were able to take the focus away from the son and see the need to develop additional coping skills. The problem was not only the son's, but was each member's. Thus, they became better able to control their own anxieties while, at the same time, improving the son's confidence level. The son also had tremendous pressure taken off him, as he was no longer the focal point of the family's expectations. This enabled him to concentrate on learning new ways to manage the anxiety created by his low confidence level.

The father's response to this different perception of the problem was, "You know, I was getting more upset with the problems between my wife and me than I was with my son, who I was ready to get desperate with, if you know what I mean." He became very amenable to focusing his attention on his relationship with his wife, thereby taking some pressure off his son. The father realized that the loss of control he was experiencing with his son and wife was his problem, not his son's. He also said, "It's a good thing you didn't try to tell me there was something wrong with me cause I would have gotten up and left." He was referring to a (normalizing) comment that "given the conditions, his responses were very understandable." Therefore, never assume that a family in crisis is able to understand even the simplest of dynamics. Anxiety has a way of distorting even the most basic issues.

STAGE EIGHT: Identification, Management, and Acceptance of Feelings Precipitated by the Crisis

Identification

Stage seven is basically an education process that prepares the family for the identification of the feelings that are the most unwanted or threatening to its well being. Using Figure 8.1 with the family in stage seven provides both you and the family with a tool to help identify these feelings. All that is necessary is to ask them to review these feelings and choose, first as individuals and then collectively as a family, the one feeling that is the most feared, troublesome, or unwanted.

Acceptance

Following this process each family member is polled as to their acceptance of what feeling the family fears or feels threatened by the most. Finally the family reaches a consensus as to which feeling appears to be presenting the most difficulty for them. Although there may be some differences of opinion here, most families can arrive at a temporary decision about which feeling they must first attempt to manage better.

Management

The techniques for managing this most threatening feeling will actually be identified in stage ten, but clarifying the importance of finding a way to manage that most threatening feeling can be emphasized at this time. The single most critical question to ask regarding the chosen feeling is, "What does this feeling, when it's at its worst, make you want to do?" The answer to this question will provide further insight into a family's potential for self-destructive behavior, and will also allow for an additional brief assessment related to the previous acting out of this behavior, the outcome of this episode, and the degree to which the individual feels that he or she may lose control and again engage in that behavior. Remember, you can only determine the potential for self-destructive behavior and attempt to engage solutions to prevent it. Rarely can you predict whether or when it may occur.

We all tend to conceal the real extent of our vulnerability. In the family setting the answers to this question by some individuals often surprise other members and can help to sensitize them about how seriously their spouse, parent, sibling, son, or daughter is affected by this crisis.

The single most critical response related to the management of feelings is, "Your response is certainly understandable given what you are feeling and I am glad you could share it, but this is a feeling you do not have to act on. There are less destructive ways to remove the feeling you are having. Can you agree that during the next few weeks you will not engage in that behavior, and will let me know when you do feel like you might have no other choice?" Such an agreement can usually be reached. This contract offers a form of control for situations where behaviors could be threatening and/or seriously self-defeating. If an agreement cannot be reached, that individual or family is telling you that the risk factor is too high, and that they do not perceive you to have the resources available to keep them from losing control. This nonagreement necessitates an immediate referral for a more intensive evaluation. If this is the case, the intervention, except for the arranging for the immediate evaluation, is basically concluded, on a note (one would hope) of support and respect, and with a promise to provide continued support in whatever way is possible. A family's acceptance of the suggestion to view aspects of their crisis differently allows you to move into the next stage of intervention.

9

Intervention Stages
Nine through Twelve

STAGE NINE: Engaging the Family
in the Problem-Solving Process

Barring a referral to an outside source for immediate evaluation, or the determination of the need for life protecting
measures, such as hospitalization and/or intensive treatment
involving a psychiatric focus, the family is ready to examine
the problem-solving process that you are going to explain
and ask them to agree to use. Next to the educational process
in stages seven and eight, the problem-solving process is the
most essential procedure for the reaching of a healthy resolution of the crisis.

The Problem-Solving Process

The suggested problem-solving model demands family participation and agreement as solutions are developed. The
process is designed not only to identify a variety of ways to
resolve a crisis, but also to empower the family and equip
them with problem-solving skills that they can easily call on
when future crises arise. It is a prevention model, in that no
solution is agreed upon until the possible consequences of

that solution are fully examined and the skills needed to
implement the solution are rehearsed and practiced. With this
model, therefore, families and/or individuals are better prepared for what they can expect in the way of possible barriers,
difficulties in implementation and the possible risk factors
that may emerge as a result of implementation.

This process is seldom fully utilized by helping professionals because it calls upon them to take an assertive role, to be
decisive, and to struggle along with those in crisis in their
attempts to reach a mutually agreeable plan of action. Depending upon the family system the role of the intervenor
may be more authoritative than participatory or possibly
some combination of these two styles. The problem-solving
model is essential in a crisis situation because it gives the
family in crisis the structure it needs to minimize its members'
anxiety and loss of control. The importance of such a structure has been discussed in previous chapters. The problem-
solving process now becomes the vehicle for the tying
together of all of the information obtained about and the
preparations given to the family in the previous stages.

Presenting the Problem-Solving Process

Before asking the family to agree to engage in this process it is
important to briefly educate them as to its importance. The
following points need to be reviewed with them before actually presenting the model to them. They are written in first
person and can be, if you wish, communicated as they are
written.

1. The worse possible reactions to a crisis are either to do
nothing or to act on decisions or potential solutions without
giving them plenty of thought. Inactivity increases our anxiety, fear, and sense of powerlessness, while acting out of
panic usually creates new crises for us. With this in mind I am
going to present you with a problem-solving process that can
help us arrive at some immediate actions that you can take to
alleviate some of your fears and reduce some of the tension
you're now experiencing. It will also help us arrive at more

substantial decisions, which ultimately will help support the more complicated issues.

2. The solutions we arrive at may look very good here in the office but fail miserably when you try to implement them at home. If this occurs, and it will with some of our choices, remember that it does not mean that there is something wrong with you, but rather that our choice simply did not fit the problem.

3. In order for us to ensure that the odds for success are in your favor you will need to participate in the problem-solving process, and, as a family, agree to support the trying of the solution arrived at, even though some members may not necessarily agree that it is worth trying. If it doesn't work we have all learned what doesn't work. If it does work, those who did not believe it was worthwhile will learn that there are often several ways to solve a problem.

4. Finally, there are several attitudes about your current crisis that I want you to seriously consider believing in and supporting during the next few weeks. These attitudes are:

a. Every problem may now seem overwhelming, but each presents new possibilities for us to feel better about ourselves and actually become smarter and stronger.

b. No condition determines what kind of person we become or what kind of future we can have. It is how we choose to respond to our conditions or crises that determines our future.

c. Not all crisis situations or the conditions that bring them on can be changed, but there are always ways we can take control of such a situation so that we do not become its victim.

d. Even though you may not believe it of yourself or of one another, each one of you has something intensely valuable to offer your family toward the solving of this crisis, and the individual problems that the crisis is creating.

e. Life simply does not care who you are. It does not care if you're the smartest member of the family, the strongest member, the best looking, or the most talented. You are going to be faced with very difficult and painful conditions at times, and at other times enjoy happiness and contentment. If you understand this fact of life you will also understand that crises do not last forever. The opportunity to feel good about your life will come your way again and you can speed up this process by asking for help. To ask for and accept help in no way means that you are a failure or incompetent. It is very wise to understand that no one person has all the answers, and that we (you) need one another.

f. Finally, you must be willing to take some risks. No one is born successful. Achieving success takes the ability to fail frequently and to learn from these failures about what doesn't work, what you don't like, and what you must do next. You must see any failure as moving you one step closer to success. You must be willing to take some risks, and perhaps to try some things that may make you feel uncomfortable, if you are going to find your way to a happier life. You may be asked to take these risks as part of the solution we decide to try. They will help us learn what's going to lead to the successful resolution of this crisis.

At this point, present the problem-solving process to the family. (Figure 9.1). Ask them to briefly review the drawing with you and whether they have any questions. Briefly explain the diagram to them, and then move on to stage ten.

STAGE TEN: Identifying and Selecting the Problem— Determining and Accepting the Solutions

Seven Steps in Identification and Selection

This stage can be broken down into the following seven steps:

1. The major problems facing the family have already been identified and discussed. Agreement, however, must be reached as to which of those problems presents the most immediate threat. Using the problem-solving process, and

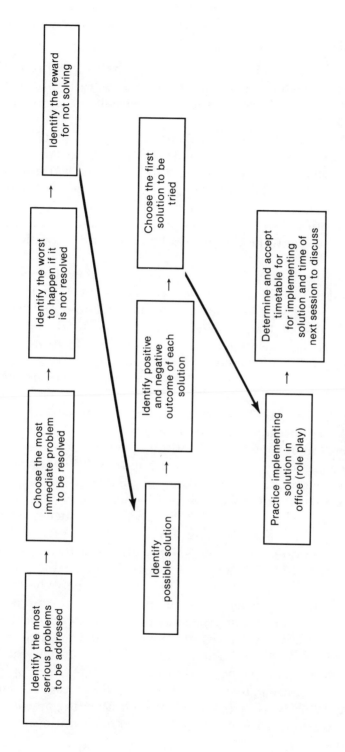

FIGURE 9.1. Problem-solving chart.

visual aids such as a blackboard, have the family list the major problems identified earlier. Help them with this process, and remind them when necessary of issues (losses) you have discussed.

2. This step will be more difficult. It will necessitate your using both processing skills and assertiveness to keep the focus on what has been determined to be the major threat to this family. Have the family members attempt to prioritize their problems, from the most threatening to the least. In some situations two areas may present the same potential threat. If so, continue the process by determining solutions for each.

3. Ask the family to describe the worst they fear will happen if this problem is not resolved. Denial may "kick in" at this time. It will need to be confronted. Those in crisis, generally out of fear, tend to minimize potential danger, thereby placing themselves at greater risk. The denial of danger prohibits the taking of the appropriate preventive and/or protective measures. This step serves to motivate the family to seek a resolution.

4. In this step you'll be asking a question that most people are startled by because they have never entertained the concept that there can be a reward for continuing self-defeating behavior. The question to be asked of the family is, "What do you think is the reward for not solving this problem?"

Do you recall our discussion in Chapter 2 about the purpose of self-defeating behavior? When we are threatened, and the coping skills available to us do not work, we grab on to whatever promises to work. If lying successfully keeps us from being punished, and a threat is diminished, we are relieved and the next time we are threatened we lie. Whatever makes us feel safe we tend to do again and again. It is important for this family to understand that their own self-defeating or self-destructive behaviors are utilized and repeated because they remove the threat facing them. All it means when these behaviors are being used is that the family is simply unaware of what else they can do to remove the threat without placing themselves in jeopardy or in a self-defeating position. Once this is understood, you are ready to move on to step 5.

5. During this step you can suggest possibilities, but also encourage family members to share what they believe will work. All suggestions are acceptable and should be listed on the board to help in the move to step 6.

6. Every solution has positive as well as negative consequences. It is important to examine each solution for the possible positive and negative outcomes and list these next to each solution. When families can see these possible outcomes they are better able to choose which risks they are willing to take. One solution, for instance, may have ten positive and only three negative outcomes, but despite the abundance of positive consequences the family may choose to eliminate this solution because one of the possible negative outcomes is more than they are willing to risk. It also works the other way. One strongly positive outcome can seem worth the risk of having to deal with several negative outcomes. Once this step has been completed and the reason for it explained, move on to step 7.

7. This step is another prioritizing process. It calls for a consensus as to what is to be tried first, and if it fails, what is to be tried next, and so on. Once the priority has been established, move on to stage eleven.

Possible Interventions with Emergency Situations

If you have reached this stage and are still addressing level 1 and 2 concerns (as discussed in Chapter 7 under stage six), there are several interventions that must be employed.

1. Contact support systems.
2. Arrange for daily contact with the youth as often as is necessary until he or she has regained balance (resolved the crisis).
3. Discuss with the youth how to manage day to day, solutions to attempt, activities to engage in at school, etc.
4. Link the youth with 24-hour crisis centers should the situation escalate after school hours.
5. Request outside evaluation and/or outside counseling.

6. Transport the youth or request transport to an emergency facility if the danger is imminent or an medical emergency also exists (see also the legal considerations in Chapter 10).

STAGE ELEVEN: Setting the Time Table and Rehearsing the Chosen Solution

Because of the short term duration of the crisis state and the need to take immediate action it is important to arrive at solutions that the family can be immediately implement, in part or fully, upon leaving the office. Delays will only allow the family's anxiety to intensify and further block a healthy resolution. Solutions, therefore, ought to be implemented within 24 hours after the interview, and several solutions should be available for implementation if more than one day passes before the next appointment.

Finally, never send a family home with a solution that has not been rehearsed in the office. Role playing is very beneficial, as it will identify those barriers that might defeat their efforts. Practicing how to avoid these barriers can be very valuable. Furthermore, role playing can build confidence and further minimize the anxiety that trying anything new (risk) is going to create, because it helps to define the specific skills or activities that the individual has available to manage the more difficult aspects of the solution.

This process will demand assertiveness on the part of the intervenor. He/she will need to insert the possible barriers that might arise, take on an antagonistic role, if necessary, as well as model positive responses to the difficult problems that the family might encounter. This is difficult for many beginning intervenors because it puts them on the proverbial "hot seat." The family, in other words, becomes the judge of whether the intervenor is being helpful. This stage actually completes the problem-solving process and allows the intervenor to move to the final intervention process, stage twelve.

STAGE TWELVE: Reassessing the Family Status

The family has now been given the best you have to offer. However, not all of your efforts will have had an impact. Fear creates a reluctance to entertain new thoughts or new solutions. It becomes important, therefore, to determine if the family now feels more hopeful and in control than when they first sat down in the office. Ask them directly if they feel better and/or more hopeful. If they do not, then you must assess whether you have actually done all you can. They may need additional time so that their discomfort can be reduced and not prohibit their implementing your recommendations, or a referral way be necessary.

This is a judgment only you as the intervenor can make. You have been exposed to the emotional intensity expressed by the family, to their level of ability to work with and digest the cognitive material, and to their level of acceptance of or resistance to the entire process. By the time you have moved through the previous stages you are likely to have a fairly good sense of the ability of this family to complete the intervention process, stabilize, and resolve their crisis.

Remember, the primary goal of crisis intervention is to return the family to their level of functioning prior to the crisis. If they can seize the opportunities presented by a crisis they can achieve a higher level of functioning, but while this can and does sometimes occur, you should not minimize the success you have achieved if you have at least helped the family to return to their previous level of functioning.

SUMMARY

These twelve stages of intervention will be utilized in each interview as new information and issues emerge during the family's pursuit of the recommended solutions. Some stages may consume more time and attention than others, but each stage needs to be addressed in each interview. The process never changes, only its area of focus. One session may be mostly problem-solving while another may stress redefining the issues.

You now have the information and tools needed to engage and assist families in crisis. Certain issues, such as suicide, violence, or sexual preference may demand your seeking additional training to increase both your ability to talk intelligently about these issues, and the appropriateness of your assessments and recommended interventions. The crisis intervention process, however, can be used across all issues.

Chapter 10 will provide a brief introduction to several emerging issues facing today's families and schools. Training in these areas can be provided by the authors at the Institute for Trauma and Loss in Children, 2051 West Grand Boulevard, Detroit, MI 48208.

You will also find in the Appendix a stage-by-stage summary of the questions, statements, and tools that have been discussed. At this point all you need to do is to take a risk, use the knowledge and tools we have provided, and find what fits best with your style, personality, skills, and experience. We would like to hear about your experiences and will respond to your questions, so please write us at the above address.

III

SPECIAL CONSIDERATIONS

10

Grief:
Family Related Issues

James Couillard*

A family system responds no differently to a trauma or loss than an individual. It moves through the various stages and exhibits many of the same grief reactions. There are, however, additional crises precipitated when a family experiences a traumatic event and/or the loss of one of its members.

The family is a system. This system has developed roles, responsibilities, relationships, alignments, and specific ways for managing conflict and dealing with problems. It is systematic in the way that it functions. In a crisis the family as a system will either open itself up to outside help (when they can no longer resolve their difficulties), or, as a system, it will close down, become more rigid, and withdraw from or refuse any offer of help.**

---

*James Couillard, M.A., is a school counsellor whose area of expertise is in group work with children of divorce as well as substance abuse and chemical dependency in children.

**This difference can be crucial. For example, at a time of grief, the open family system will manage much better and develop fewer chronic or pathological reactions to trauma or loss than will a closed family.

Imagine a family of four. They are doing well. There are no major problems. Everyone was happy when mom became pregnant, and the child was born healthy. We now have a family of five. What happens? This family's systematic way of relating and surviving is going to have to change. Now that there is a new infant in the house, mom's relationships with her other children and her husband change just from the fact of her needing the time to care for the baby. The children may also be expected to take on some additional responsibilities. As mom's time with them decreases they must turn to one another. Dad may need to work longer hours to support the family. He also at times may have to "fill-in" for mom with the older children.

This system has changed. The roles, relationships, and expectations are now different, and the change has brought on new challenges and new crises. The system may do well, even with the changes it must make, but there will be periods of conflict and even loss reactions because this system, the family, is no longer the same (Steele, in press).

The addition of a member to a family can and usually does alter the family as a system. There may be resulting crises, but these are usually manageable. The system stabilizes and many of its patterns remain. When the same system, however, loses one of its members, it can change drastically and may never reestablish itself. After a loss or a traumatic event family systems can be at risk (Steele, in press).

RISK FACTORS

"The more emotionally important the deceased family member, the greater the impact on the family. The more emotionally dependent the survivors, the greater the likelihood of future trouble, as the shock wave ripples through the generations" (Dopson, 1983, p. 208).

When a family loses its major caretaker it must not only deal with the loss of that person, but now must also struggle to find another source for its physical, emotional, and even financial support. Their grief, therefore, is compounded by the anxiety of not knowing how this might be accomplished.

When a family loses a child the grief of the parent(s) will of course be intense, perhaps so intense that the grieving parent will be unable physically or emotionally to care for the surviving members, especially the surviving children. The system is often devastated. The surviving children have not only lost someone close to them. They have also lost the comforting, consistent, and familiar interaction of that grieving parent. The longer the parent remains depressed, the greater the risk that the surviving children will develop pathological symptoms. This type of loss is particularly devastating to parents who saw their child as an extension of themselves. It is not unusual for fathers, for example, who have been close to their only son and then lose that son, to distance themselves so much and for so long from the surviving family members that the family system becomes dysfunctional and even destroyed.

Therefore, such families need a great deal of help dealing with their grief from extended family members and friends. The more limited these resources, the higher the risk that the family may become dysfunctional and not survive. The family system that closes itself off to outside help is only compounding its grief and worsening the crises that will develop as a result.

WHAT GRIEVING FAMILIES NEED

1. Grieving families need outside help from relatives and friends.

2. Grieving families need someone who can temporarily assume the daily adult responsibilities, so that the surviving parents can have time to grieve while knowing that their surviving children are being provided for.

3. Grieving families need someone to help them process their most frightening thoughts and feelings, which, while quite normal, may include attacking and blaming other family members.

4. Grieving families need to see the support of friends who attend the memorial service, the family gathering after the burial, or who drop by the house periodically and help in

little but caring ways, such as bringing over food dishes or watching the children so that the grieving parents can be alone for awhile and not have to worry about upsetting their children (with their crying, etc).

5. Grieving families need information about the grief process, as well as about resources they can utilize as needed.

6. Grieving families will need people around them who are comfortable talking about the loss, who acknowledge their pain rather than try to limit it, and who, when possible, have had a loss of their own and can now talk about their experience.

7. Grieving families need someone on whom they can displace their anger, pain, and frustration, someone who understands these reactions and does not take them personally, and who remains available as a friend when the family is able to let them be there for them.

Not everyone has the experience, the knowledge, or the energy to be a friend to the family in these ways. Helping individuals through their grief is never easy, and it is even more difficult to help families through their grief. There are probably many more professionals capable of working effectively with individuals than there are those able to work effectively with families. Don't be afraid to enlist the aid of organizations and individuals who specialize in working with families.

TEEN SUICIDE AND THE CONTAGION EFFECT

The following is an anecdotal account as told to the author of an actual situation concerning the suicide of a student, the subsequent reactions of other students following this loss, and its impact on the school counselor.

Anecdote

Fifty-two kids. This is Easter vacation, and there have already been fifty-two students for whom we've had to do interventions since the suicide of one of our students. Let's see. . . .

Fifty-two out of eight hundred is 6.5%. That doesn't sound bad. Unless you consider the *one*. You know the one . . . the one we did not do an intervention on . . . the one who died, and who might have lived had we known. Then maybe, just maybe, there might not have been all these others.

I was, ironically, at a workshop on teen suicide when our secretary called and informed me that one of our students had been found, hanged, in his garage the previous evening. It was too close to dismissal for me to get back to school in time to see the several students who had come to the counseling office to talk, and so all I could do was to try and gather my thoughts and deal with my own shocked disbelief that this had happened. The abstract concept we had been studying in the workshop had been translated into the real kick in the gut of losing someone you know and care for.

That night, as I lay awake wondering what to do and trying to make sense of what happened, I searched my memory for thoughts of Ryan [pseudonym], the thirteen-year-old boy who now lay comatose in a nearby hospital. An eighth-grader, Ryan was a good looking boy, an athlete who wasn't wild about academics, but who reveled in the chaotic social life of a suburban junior high school. Ryan was in a special education program for learning disabled kids, but his class work was always a struggle for him.

The fact was, I didn't know Ryan that well. He had been in a few times to see me in seventh grade. I remembered changing his schedule once and helping solve a conflict with some other students at another time, but nothing remarkable. Just an "average" kid, whatever that is. So what happened?

As is often the case in these situations, no one but God and Ryan will ever know. The external circumstances certainly gave no clue that Ryan was predisposed to suicide. He was just finishing a successful baseball season and was looking forward to going bow hunting with his father. He excused himself from the dinner table that evening and went into the yard to practice shooting his bow at a target behind the garage. Inside the garage was a rope harness attached to the rafters and designed to hold the deer both Ryan and his dad hoped they would "bag" during their forthcoming hunting trip. This is where they found Ryan hanging a few hours later. He was rushed to a nearby hospital where he lay tethered to a life-support system. He would hang on to life one more week before the final decision was made to let him go.

It wasn't clear then and it will never be clear what exactly happened. Ryan's father told me that he thought Ryan might have been going through the motions of a successful deer hunt. After he "shot" his deer with his bow and arrow behind the garage, he was pretending to haul it inside the garage and hoist it up on to the harness in the rafters. Somehow he got entangled in the ropes, or maybe he was just curious about what it would feel like to have the rope around his neck, or to hang like the deer he had just shot or . . . speculation was fruitless. The inescapable fact, like a huge black cloud enveloping those who knew him, was that Ryan was gone.

All of my training and 20 years of experience working with adolescents did not prepare me for what was to happen in school during the days subsequent to the tragedy. Word of Ryan's condition had been slow to leak out on Monday, but on Tuesday, when I returned to school, all hell broke loose. As the information spread from those close to Ryan, to kids who knew him from the various classes he was in, to his many acquaintances in both elementary and secondary school, the hysteria became almost palpable. Sobbing students were being sent to the counseling office by the dozens. Red-eyed kids wandered the halls in clusters during class time. The restrooms were filled to capacity with students crying and embracing each other.

Fortunately, the district had trained a "crises team" a few years earlier, and as a part of that team I had some idea of how to respond. Initially, though, it seemed that nothing we did could calm the emotional storm that swept the building. A team of school psychologists, social workers, my fellow counselors, and I hastily convened to decide how we should proceed. We decided that a "triage" approach, like hospitals employ in a disaster setting, would be best. We would "screen" kids for three possible treatments: individual counseling for those students hardest hit (i.e., kids who were either hysterical or at risk for self-destruction behaviors to begin with); group counseling for those who wanted it or as a means of "culling out" those who needed individual attention; and the rest of the students would either be sent home or back to class as the circumstances warranted. In this fashion we counseled closed to 75 students the first day.

As Ryan clung to life in the nearby medical facility, rumors were rampant. Kids descended upon the hospital by the dozens and some, much to our horror, succeeded in getting into the I.C.U. to see Ryan. Even now, 6 months later, we are dealing with the post-traumatic stress of those kids who saw their friend tethered to the life support systems, pale, comatose, and, for all intents and purposes, lifeless. One girl swore he squeezed her hand in recognition. Another said his eyes followed her as she walked around to "pull the plug." As these accounts filtered back to school during the rest of the week, waves of students would descend upon the counseling office, their emotions cranked up or down in sync with the latest rumor. Ryan didn't just die once during that week. He died and came back to life several times, as we all rode an emotional roller coaster fueled by the electric atmosphere that only junior high emotions can generate.

We soon realized that we were powerless to control the events of the next few days. We tried to set up a "rumor-control," but it was a pitiful attempt compared to the all-encompassing "grapevine" already operating among the 800 students of this junior high. We asked, begged, and cajoled the students *not* to visit the hospital. Even Ryan's family could not keep the kids from keeping a "vigil" in the lobby and sneaking up to I.C.U. whenever the security guard turned his back.

Inevitably, some adolescents (true to form) handled the event with the callousness that only troubled kids can show. "R-Y-A-N. If he comes back, we'll hang him again!" they were heard to chant in the hallways. The ensuing fights resulted in suspensions and added even more tension to the already overcharged atmosphere.

Somehow our best efforts did not seem to be strong enough to stem the tide. We met with parents and staff after school. We had an "open door" policy for any kid needing help. The professional resources of our school district, one of the largest school districts in the state, were at our disposal—yet, somehow we were powerless to deal with the emotional freight train that was still careening out of control.

When they finally disconnected the life-support system and Ryan passed away, it seemed almost anticlimatic. Many students had already been through the grieving processes of denial, shock, anger, and depression several times. Now they were emotionally drained, washed-out, and weak, like survivors of a shipwreck finally cast upon a beach somewhere remote and inaccessible. They were, above all, vulnerable.

In the weeks that followed the funeral several students had to be closely monitored for severe depression and intrusive suicidal ideations. We were especially worried about one girl in particular—Gina. She had been Ryan's "steady" girlfriend off and on for the past few months, but at the time of his death their relationship had been "off." Because the break up had been at her insistence, and because Ryan was allegedly upset as a result of Gina's rejection of him, she wholeheartedly blamed herself for his death. She wandered the halls in a zombie-like state, refusing to talk or make eye contact with anyone and compulsively clutching a worn picture of her and Ryan. A few days after the funeral we had to rush her to the hospital because she had taken an overdose of aspirin. Her mother steadfastly refused to follow our recommendation that Gina be hospitalized. Although she received outside therapy, her condition did not improve. A few weeks later she was caught with a bag full of aspirin in yet another planned attempt. Her mother still refused placement in a psychiatric treatment center.

What was particularly worrisome about Gina's attempts was the fact that she was one of the most popular kids in the school. An "all-A" student, star athlete, and acknowledged leader, Gina was everybody's idea of "the perfect child." Because she was a role model for other students, her deep depression and suicidal actions were very disturbing. Whether or not Ryan's death was a suicide, Gina's attempts were bona fide. In a sense, her actions made suicide a legitimate mode of problem solving for the other kids in the school. They looked up to (in some cases almost worshipped) her, and she was getting a lot of attention for her actions.

Currently it seems as if the school is a war zone. The enemy is invisible, cunning, and indestructible. The students are like veterans of some mysterious warfare, many suffering from post-traumatic stress syndrome. Subsequent to Ryan's death we have had to hospitalize ten kids for serious depression and/or for suicide attempts. All together we have had to conduct 52 interventions on kids who were either contemplating suicide or depressed enough for someone to be seriously concerned about them. Thus far this year a week has not gone by when we haven't had to refer a student to assessment for possible suicidal behaviors. Sometimes there are as many as two a day.

The obvious question is "why?" Why is it that there are so many depressed kids in one school? Why are they trying to kill themselves? Is there anything we can do? The answers to these questions are, of course, complex. The best we can do is to speculate. Part of the reason for the unusually high number of suicidal kids in our school has to be because of Ryan's death. At least 24 of the interventions we have done have been with kids identified as friends of Ryan. In a sense these kids were doubly traumatized, in that a year and a half earlier one of their elementary school classmates had been killed by a car while crossing a busy street. In counseling many brought up this tragedy in conjunction with Ryan's death.

Maybe the large number of interventions are also a result of our becoming more sophisticated in terms of identifying and dealing with teen depression. Thanks in large part to the pioneering work done by Bill Steele in training educators to deal with teen suicide, many of us now know what questions to ask and what to do when confronted with traumatized kids. In retrospect, I shudder to think what might have happened had we *not* been trained to deal with this situation. One can't help but speculate that we might have lost one or more of the other kids if we hadn't intervened so effectively. Perhaps a look at how we intervened, at what "worked" and what didn't "work," might be of some benefit to those of you who, God forbid, have to deal with a similar disaster.

In his *Developing Crisis Response Teams in Schools* (in press) Steele suggests a variety of guidelines for schools to utilize in responding to a student's death. A retrospective look at those suggestions and how they worked or didn't work with our students might help us to understand why so many kids at our school required interventions, and why our interventions were successful.

Steele suggests that crisis team members should be in the classroom when the announcement of the tragedy is made. Because of the "grapevine" effect, however, students knew about Ryan before a "formal" announcement could be made. Furthermore, our crisis team members had their hands full with the large number of kids who frequented the "drop in" center in the counseling area. It could be speculated that the "individual" way that the news was broken to most of the students might have precipitated some of the students' crises, and that a number of these might have been averted if that aspect of the tragedy could have been controlled. The staff also had little time, unfortunately, to discuss the tragedy in Ryan's classes. Although we made ourselves available and the teachers did an admirable job of handling classroom grief, this aspect of the event probably could have received more systematic treatment. Regrettably, the staff was limited in time and resources, and therefore had to deal with the numerous kids in crisis in the counseling center. We probably could have used some more help in the classrooms.

Furthermore, "the conspiracy of silence" Steele refers to in his text was evident in the classrooms we did visit. It was as if saying anything was almost a betrayal of Ryan. This situation obviously made the teacher and the crisis counselor less inclined to pursue the topic. If we had it to do again we would go into the classes with a prepared "lesson plan" on grief, and thus would be ready if the kids were not talking. We would know, as Steele says, that "this silence is a defense against an overwhelming upheaval of feelings that seem to be on the verge of going out of control."

A related aspect of this tragedy that deserves further exploration was the reaction of the teaching staff. Although an initial meeting was well-attended, subsequent meetings had to be canceled due to a lack of attendance. It was almost as if "the conspiracy of silence" extended to the staff as well as the students, and that there was a unanimous agreement that the tragedy would go away faster if it was just not talked about. This staff, however, had already been heavily traumatized by suicide. A teacher had died by suicide several years earlier, and two staff members had lost sons to suicide. This type of death, therefore, was presumably a very difficult topic for the teachers to discuss in as well as outside the classroom. Therefore it was probably *doubly* important for us to provide organized classroom support, since it was certainly very painful for many of these teachers to deal with this topic in a classroom setting. Furthermore, we probably should have had "lesson plans" for our staff presentations to help beat "the conspiracy." Teachers, however, can be the most difficult group to teach.

Also in retrospect, we had no clear expectations as to how long the crisis team should remain in the building. Thus, when the funeral was over, the respective team members went back to their own building. This was probably a mistake, because those few of us left with the students were unable to meet adequately the needs of the many hurting kids at the school. Although we continued to conduct grief support groups and to intervene on an individual basis, those of us involved in the process were (are!) bordering on "burnout." Perhaps a prolonged "assault" by trained professionals might have averted some of the subsequent suicide attempts. Certainly, the large number of interventions required indicates the need for additional support.

In conclusion, it could be said that 6 months later the crisis is not over. It has just entered a new stage. This new stage, however, is every bit as dangerous and unpredictable as the initial crisis we faced when Ryan died. It is characterized by a high level of suicidal ideations, feelings of abandonment, and "acting out" behaviors in and out of school by Ryan's friends and acquaintances. All indications are that we can probably

expect at least one more year of increased risk among the
student body in terms of suicidal thoughts and actions. Hope-
fully, we'll maintain our vigilance and avert yet another disaster.

*   *   *

The above anecdotal account describes a reality that many
schools have experienced. Loss, especially by suicide, can
precipitate chaos in a school setting. If intervention to prevent subsequent attempts is to be successful, we must first
understand how grief after a suicide is different from grief
after natural death. Such information is also critical to the
development of policies and procedures related to the
(school's) organized response to the surviving student body.

Families after a Loss

Suicide not only affects students and school staff, but also
raises many questions related to helping surviving families.
Steele and Leonhardi (1986) and Steele (in press) provide very
practical information related to the survivor grief of family
members and fellow students, the intervention needs of both
groups, and critical policies and procedures related to a
school response to a student's suicide.

Grief after a suicide death is different than the grief experienced after a death by natural causes. A sudden, unantici-
pated death precipitates a response different from the response to an anticipated death. A violent death, such as a
murder, involves different issues than a nonviolent death.
Knowing the basic differences between the types of grief that
follow these different forms of death is important when intervening with families. Such knowledge can help in assessing
the potential risk factors that can emerge in the survivors, as
well as in determining the most appropriate interventions.

After a suicide family members must contend with the
following issues. These are generally not present following
other forms of death, and if they are, present themselves
differently.

A Chosen Act

The act of suicide reflects a sense of hopelessness about life. It is as if the deceased said to the survivor, "You cannot help me. You failed me."

Guilt: The guilt of a survivor is long-term and massive. Survivors frequently see themselves as being responsible.

Unexplained act: The guilt of a survivor is intensified by the question "why?" An accident, murder, or illness allows survivors to focus their grief. After a suicide there is no place to focus grief except on failure.

Stigma: The public's response to a suicide, although changing, is still one of blame, or of a questioning of the family's ability to be loving and caring, thereby further intensifying the survivors' guilt and alienating them from much needed support.

Taboo: Suicide is still an act few wish to talk about, even among surviving family members, relatives, and close friends. The less the survivors and those who know the surviving family members talk about it, the more alienated and isolated the family becomes and the less opportunity they have to work through their grief. This "closed" response precipitates many subsequent, and often devastating, problems for family members.

Violence: Suicide is a violent death, and as such leaves the surviving family members with violent images, dreams, day mares, and intense pain.

Legacy: After a suicide it is not unusual to discover that the thought of suicide is being entertained by a surviving family member or close friend. Suicide can precipitate a "contagious-like" response, as schools all too painfully know.

As can be seen, these differences alone will dictate some interventions that are different from the interventions used after other forms of death. Space simply does not provide for adequate coverage, and we again refer the reader to other resources, especially Steele and Leonhardi (1986) and Steele (in press).

When the suicide of a student takes place the school can best serve the families of the surviving students by providing an assembly for these families to talk to counselors and teachers about the issues related to suicide. They are frequently fearful about the risk to their own children after such a tragedy and certainly need to know what to look for and do should they suspect their youth is suicidal. It is also important at such an assembly to educate them as to the differences in grief after a suicide simply because some members of that audience, perhaps unknown to you, may have had experience with a suicide in their own family or circle of friends. These people need to have this information to bring closure to their own grief. Educating families about these issues can be a very effective intervention after a suicide, and is a service that we should expect our schools to provide.

The following guidelines are taken from *Survivors: After a Suicide What Can We Do?* (Steele & Leonhardi, 1986). They are intended to aid the counselor who is to meet with the family members of suicide victims.

GENERAL GUIDELINES

• Initiate a conversation about the suicide, and let them know that their grief is different from the grief brought on by a death by natural causes. Do not be afraid to use the word suicide; doing so helps to desensitize the family, and also helps them to face the reality of what happened. Encourage the family to have a personalized funeral or memorial service and not to "hush it up," even though they may be uncomfortable about it.

• Do not say "I understand" because surviving families will not believe you unless you too are a survivor. However, listening to them talk without being judgmental is very helpful. Listening conveys to them that you do not see them as terrible people, which they may feel that they are.

• Let the survivors know that although they may feel guilty, the death was not their fault. They did not make the choice. It is helpful to repeat this.

• Share any information about other suicides in the community or in your personal life. Survivors may feel less shame when reminded that they are not the only ones to have had this experience.

• Provide literature about suicide and grief.

• Give the survivors permission to feel angry at the deceased, to cry, to be relieved, and to experience *all* of their emotions.

• Inform the survivor about the major stress that he or she is and will be experiencing. Encourage survivors to be kind to themselves, to eat well, and to get plenty of sleep (although all of these will probably be very difficult).

• Do not try to answer the question "Why?". Survivors will ask it over and over, and finally will answer some parts of the question in their own minds, but this question can never be fully answered.

• After a suicide the survivors feel that everything is out of control. Encourage them to reestablish their daily routines so they can begin to feel a little more in control.

• Recognize that survivors are often angry at what happened and that they may take it out on you. They are not angry at you. Be understanding!

• Provide information about what support groups are available and encourage their use. (Call you local suicide prevention center.)

• If possible, sponsor educational programs about suicide and encourage the survivors to attend.

• Sometimes the survivors become suicidal themselves. Watch for the clues, and do not be afraid to ask them about how bad they are feeling, and/or if they are having thoughts about dying and/or suicide.

• Support any religious convictions that the survivors may have, but remember that their faith may be shaken. They are not bad people if they temporarily lose interest in God. They may regain their faith later on.

• Inform the survivors about the grief process that they may experience. In the early hours, days, and weeks after the death it may often appear that the survivors are unable to absorb any information or advice that you may provide. But survivors report that this early information is helpful, and *that repetition is also useful.* No information can erase the pain or shorten the normal grief process, but sometimes it can help survivors to be more understanding and accepting of themselves as they experience their intense grief.

Summary

Grief after a suicide is different from grief after a natural death. Intervention for survivors after a suicide has a distinct focus because of these differences, and therefore understanding all of the similarities and disparities is critical to the intervenor's effectiveness and ability to assist survivors. The resources listed at the end of this chapter can help to better one's understanding of these differences.

AFTER A HOMICIDE

The grief after a murder is complicated by numerous factors. The murder of a parent, sibling, relative, loved one, friend, or acquaintance—each of these can bring about a different reaction, in addition to the common responses. What kind of murder was it—vehicular homicide, murder accompanied by sexual assault, by torture, preceded by a kidnapping, or succeeded by a violation of the body? Who was the assailant—a parent, sibling, relative, stranger? Steele (in press) refers to a number of the considerations related to the grief suffered by the survivors after a homicide.

The attributes of the victim also affect the nature of the grief. It is sad but when an infant is killed, others are empathetic but rarely outraged. "You can always have another baby." is a comment that reflects this society's view of such a tragic and violent loss. The grief, as well as any support for the survivors in this situation, is frequently minimized by such attitudes. The death of an older person is seldom taken as seriously as that of a young person. "They lived their life." reflects an attitude that is certainly less than supportive. Forgotten is the violent way in which this life ended.

If the victim is gay or lesbian the responses can again be less than supportive. In some situations this is the first time that the life style of the victim has been revealed. This intensifies the grief for the survivors. Even if this was public knowledge, however, the survivors may not be treated by the criminal justice system in the same way that the survivors of heterosexual victims are treated. Indeed, the criminal justice system can bring untold grief to any and all survivors simply because of the prolonged period of time it frequently takes for the courts to do their work. Also coming in to play here are issues such as plea bargaining, insanity, the sentencing process, testifying, and media coverage. For some this involvement with the justice system brings about the displacement of their energies into a fight for justice. This delays the grief process until the trial is over. These emotions then break loose and, rather than relief, the end of the trial brings the long suppressed grief to the surface.

Siblings

The siblings of children who are murdered are often forgotten. The myth that children do not grieve or cannot understand death still exists for many adults. Surviving children may be terrified of being abandoned or left alone, or they may fear that the same thing is now going to happen to them. Depending upon their age, they may not understand the permanency of death. Friends and schoolmates can actually make things worse, as they may, out of their own uneasiness, make fun of what happened. Their role in the family may also change. A child may suddenly become the only child, or the oldest child, or the only male or female child as a result of the murder. Such a change can create increased anxiety. "At times they may attempt to take over the identity of the murdered child in order to ease their parents' grief" (*NOVA Bulletin*, 1985, p. 2).

Surviving parents are frequently in such pain they have little left with which to nurture their other children. In fact, it is not unusual for parents to communicate that they expect their other children not to present them with any demands during this time. This can serve to intensify the sense of abandonment that a sibling feels, and can intensify an anger, that will, in time, turn to resentment. The lives of the surviving children are ultimately disrupted in every way, and if their grief is not attended to by parents and/or friends, it could pave the way for fear, anxiety, anger, and mistrust, all of which can lead to seriously dysfunctional behavior at a later date.

Witness to Murder

The number of incidents in which children witness the murder of their own parent is growing. In 1981, of 2,000 homicides in Los Angeles County, about 10% involved children as witnesses (Zeanah & Burk, 1984). For many of the reasons cited earlier few of these children are referred for treatment. However, the recent acknowledgment by the psychiatric profession that young children do experience depression has prompted new studies of children who are witnesses to their parent's murder.

Anxiety, hyperactivity, fear of being alone, sleep disturbance, and enuresis are common symptoms in young children who witness parental murder (Bergen, 1958; Schetky, 1978). Imagine also a child's ambivalence after such a trauma when he or she is asked to testify. Testifying, for example, in the case of a mother's murder by her father, a young girl experiences the conflict between telling the truth and protecting her father. The younger the child, the greater the potential for tremendous conflict. If that child is still egocentric in her thinking and harbored death wishes toward her mother, this murder might lead her to believe that her wishes had the power to make things come true, thereby adding to her terror.

It is not unusual in these situations for children, in order to remain connected to the dead parent, to over identify with the deceased. If the child has been overwhelmed by the fear of similar aggression, he or she may also identify with the aggressor. Other children may identify with the protector as a means of coping (Zeanah & Burk, 1984). These possibilities give us some insight into the complex and disturbing symptoms that can result for children who are surviving witnesses of their parent's murder.

GUIDELINES

Most children who have witnessed the murder of a parent or a sibling should be referred for assessment to specialists who specifically treat young survivors of homicide. The following is a list of considerations one should have in mind when dealing with any survivors of a homicide (*NOVA Bulletin*, 1985, p. 9). Added to these considerations is a list of the national organizations that can provide further information. Many programs are now in existence, especially in cities, and so we suggest contacting your local suicide prevention center for additional resources.

The following list of gestures and thoughts can mean a great deal to survivors as they struggle with their grief and anger.

- Allow survivors to grieve in whatever way they wish and for as long as they wish.
- Allow survivors to cry freely. It is a healthy expression of grief and releases tensions.
- Allow survivors to talk about the victim, his or her life, and the murder. Allow them to criticize the victim and to talk about both good and bad times.
- Allow survivors to get angry at you, the victim, the criminal, the criminal justice system, or simply at the unfairness of life. Anger needs expression and sharing.
- Remember the survivors and the victim at holiday time, the anniversary date of the murder, and birthdays. Let the survivors know that you remember too.
- Allow the survivors some time out occasionally from day-to-day pressures. Offer the surviving parent help with the children so that he or she can have a day off work, or a day out of the house.

- Reassure the survivors that the murder was not their fault or the victim's fault.
- Tell survivors that you are sorry that the murder happened and that it is horrible that someone killed their loved one.
- Support survivors in their effort to reconstruct a life, even (or especially) if it means a major change in their lifestyle, work, or place of residence.
- Let survivors know that you will remain their friend and that they mean a great deal to you.

Finally, survivors should be encouraged to seek additional emotional support, whether from mental health professionals or through self-help groups. They should be reassured that their feelings are normal, and that such feelings are overwhelming for most individuals.

Helpers should also bear in mind that there are other survivors of homicide victims who have lived through similar pain. Often such veterans are the most comforting sources of support that "new" survivors can receive. They have felt similar grief, intense anger, and overwhelming loss, and have faced the unanswered questions raised by what appears to be senseless violence.

Parents of Murdered Children (POMC) has chapters in most states that are composed of parents and other survivors who meet to talk about their children, their pain, their grief, and occasionally, their joys. In such groups survivors find that there are responsive ears who want to know more about the victim and the victim's life, as well as about the murder. To find out if there is a chapter in your area, contact POMC National Headquarters, 1739 Bella Vista, Cincinnati, Ohio 45237, (513) 721-LOVE or (513) 242-8025.

Families and Friends of Missing Persons and Violent Crime Victims sponsors self-help groups that deal with all sorts of crimes, but often are predominantly made up of the survivors of murder victims. Though mainly based in Washington State, they have affiliates elsewhere. To contact them, write Families and Friends, 8421 32nd Street, SW, Seattle, Washington 98126, (206) 362-1081.

Another national self-help group is The Compassionate Friend, Inc. It exists to provide support for parents who have lost a child to any type of death. In areas where POMC chapters do not exist, many parents of murdered children have found the support and strength they need in this group, which has the largest number of chapters of the groups mentioned here. To locate their local chapter, contact The Compassionate Friends National Headquarters, P.O. Box 1347, Oak Brook, Illinois 60521, (312) 323-5010, 10A.M. to 3P.M., Monday through Friday.

A self-help group for individuals whose spouse has died by any cause is They Help Each Other Spiritually (THEOS). To find the nearest chapter of this group, contact THEOS Foundation, 410 Penn Hills Mall, Pittsburgh, Pennsylvania 15235, (412) 243-4299.

For survivors of vehicular homicides caused by drunk driving, Mothers Against Drunk Driving (MADD) provides assistance and support through self-help groups and other activities. Write or call MADD, 669 Airport Freeway, Suite 310, Hurst, Texas 76053, (817) 268-MADD.

Persons who survive the murder of a gay or lesbian victim may wish to seek assistance from the Violence Project of the National Gay Task Force, 80 Fifth Avenue, #601, New York, N.Y. 10011, (212) 741-5800.

The Institute for Trauma and Loss in Children (TLC) (New Center Community Mental Health, 2051 W. Grand Blvd., Detroit, Michigan 48203) provides texts and videotapes designed for classroom use. Teacher guides are also available, along with training for schools (crisis teams) personnel.

SUDDEN UNEXPECTED DEATH: GENERAL CONCERNS

Sudden, unexpected death presents certain dynamics that are different from anticipated death situations (Steele, in press). Suicide and homicide are certainly unexpected deaths. A sudden death allows no time to prepare psychologically. "Consequently, the mourner tends to be traumatized upon hearing

the regrettable news. As a result he or she is much more likely
to remain in the impact stage (shock) for an inordinately long
time" (Miller, 1977, p. 17).

Initial Response

The initial response to those who have suddenly lost someone
have a tremendous impact on how those survivors will manage their grief. If the responses are such that they inhibit the
wide range of normal grief responses, the risk for increased
dysfunctional behavior in the survivors is significant (Parks,
1964). Those with bereavement counseling experience know
that such grief responses can at times appear pathological
when in fact they are normal. If a person's behavior is perceived to be pathological, not normal, or increases the anxiety
level of other survivors, it is not unusual to find the individual trying to inhibit these problematic responses.

What Is Normal?

Fatigue, dizziness, shortness of breath, numbness, headaches,
diarrhea, sleep loss, appetite loss, and heart palpitations are
among the common physical reactions. The inability to concentrate or to organize daily activities, denial, bewilderment,
silence, anger, hostility, guilt, self-blame, and a preoccupa-
tion with the image of the deceased are common emotional
reactions. When death is sudden the survivors can be overwhelmed by the sudden flooding of these physical and emotional reactions. This "flooding" response to a sudden death
can become very threatening and anxiety producing because
it leaves the survivor feeling out of control. A simple acknowledgment that what he or she are experiencing is normal
can help prevent dysfunctional behavior.

Cultural Differences

It is important to keep in mind that there can be cultural
factors that dictate how one grieves. Some cultures believe
that it is wrong to display feelings, while others hold that

crying is all right. Therefore, when some survivors show little reaction it does not necessarily mean that they are "handling" their grief well. This may be a conditioned or learned response. Unfortunately, the grief these individuals experience is frequently minimized because of their "calm" external response. Information as to what kinds of physical and emotional reactions these individuals may eventually experience can be very helpful.

Children

Children need to know the truth in order to prevent or reduce any fantasies or distortions that could develop (Rund & Hutzler, 1983). When the truth is not known, some children carry these distortions, and the accompanying grief, with them into adolescence and adulthood. Such unresolved grief can lead to episodes of depression (Goodstein, 1984). Adults have a tendency to want to minimize and/or alter the feelings of loss that children experience. This is a result of the misconception that it is best to shield them both from their own feelings, and from the feelings of parents and other adults regarding that loss. The open expression of feelings is helpful to children and needs to be encouraged. When adults avoid the open discussion and expression of feelings they, rather than shield the child, create an environment of apprehension and fear that leaves the child in the position of not being able to trust others (Albrizio, 1982).

Time

Sudden death creates tremendous time pressures, and therefore places urgent demands on those seen as helpers. A prepared set of procedures can be invaluable in maintaining an overall sense of stability in response to a situation that can throw students into emotional chaos, confusion, and crisis.

Children will want answers immediately. They will want to do something. This is why the time to decide how to respond to young people is before such a traumatic event takes place. Being empathetic with young people during a sudden death experience takes a good deal of focused energy. If one's available energy is being used to decide what to do administratively or environmentally, the time pressures will minimize the opportunity to give students the support they need. On that note, in a crisis situation the demands on your time will be coming from many directions; students, staff, the superintendent's office, community agencies, and the media, to identify just a few. Given the high incidence of death among young people in this country today, not being prepared beforehand concerning how each of these areas will be managed, and who will be responsible for what, is simply irresponsible.

SUMMARY

Each individual grieves in his or her own way, in his or her own time. There are certain patterns and commonalities, but there are also many differences. What is common for some is not common for others. Helping survivors to communicate their feelings and thoughts is the only way to find out if they are truly managing their grief. Behaviors can be deceiving. Survivors act the way they have been conditioned to act in the presence of death. Their true feelings and thoughts are not always reflected in their behavior. An important aspect of intervention, therefore, is to provide the support and encouragement survivors need to feel safe and comfortable enough to share their inner thoughts and feelings. This is usually necessary before a person can begin the process of recovery.

REFERENCES

Albrizio, M. (1982). The client who is bereaved. In J. Gorta & R. Partridge (Eds.), *Practice and management of psychiatric emergency care* (pp. 256–280). St. Louis: C. V. Mosby.
Bergen, M. E. (1958). The effect of severe trauma on a four-year-old child. *Psychoanalytic Study of the Child, 13*(407), 407–429.
Dopson, C., & Harper, M. B. (1983, January). Unresolved grief in the family. *American Family Physician, 27.* 207–211.

Goodstein, R. K. (1984). *Clinics in emergency medicine: Psychiatric emergencies.* New York: Churchill Livingstone.
Miller, M. (1977, June). Surviving the loss of a loved one: An inside look at bereavement counseling. *Thanatos, 2*(3), 14-18.
NOVA Bulletin. (1985, October). *2*(3), 1-11.
Parks, C. M. (1964). Recent bereavement as a cause of mental illness. *British Journal of Psychiatry, 110,* 198-204.
Rund, D. A., & Hutzler, J. C. (1983). Psychiatric emergencies associated with death. In *Emergency psychiatry* (pp. 231-241). St. Louis: C. V. Mosby.
Schetky, D. H. (1978). Preschoolers' response to murder of their mothers by their fathers: A study of four cases. *Bulletin of the American Academy of Psychiatry and the Law, 6*(45), 45-57.
Steele, W. (in press). *Developing crisis response teams in schools.* Holmes, FL: Learning Publications.
Steele, W., & Leonhardi, M. (1986). *Survivors: After a suicide what can we do?* Novato, CA: Academic Therapy Publications.
Zeanah, C. H., & Burk, G. S. (1984, January). A young child who witnessed her mother's murder: Therapeutic and legal considerations. *American Journal of Psychotherapy, 38,* 132-145.

ADDITIONAL READING

Survivors of Suicide

Bolton, Iris. *My son . . . My son . . .* Atlanta: Bolton Press, 1983.
Cleaver, V., & Cleaver, B. (1970). *Grover.* Philadelphia: Lippincott.
Coleman, W. L. (1979). *Understanding suicide.* Elgin, IL: David C. Cook.
Colgave, M., Bloomfield, H., & McWilliams, P. (1976). *How to survive the loss of a love.* New York: Bantam.
Davidson, G. (1984). *Understanding mourning.* Minneapolis: Augsburg.
Dunne, E., McIntosh, J., & Dunne-Maxim, K. (Eds.). (1987). *Suicide and its aftermath.* New York: Norton.
Giovacchini, P. (1981). *The urge to die: Why young people commit suicide.* New York: MacMillan.
Grollman, E. (1967). *Explaining death to children.* Boston: Beacon Press.

Hewett, J. (1980). *After suicide*. Philadelphia: Westminister Press.
LaShan, E. (1976). *Learning to say good-bye when a parent dies.* New York: Avon.
Lucas, C., & Seiden, H. (1988). *Silent grief.* New York: Scribner's.
Rosenfeed, L., & Prupas, M. (1984). *Left alive: After a suicide death in the family.* Springfield, IL: Charles C. Thomas.
Schaefer, D., & Lyons, C. (1956). *How do we tell the children?* New York: Newmarket Press.
Schiff, H. (1986). *Living through mourning*. New York: Penguin.
Stearns, A. (1984). *Living through personal crisis.* New York: Ballantine.
Steele, W. (in press). *Developing crisis response teams in schools.* Holmes, FL: Learning Publications.
Stone, H. (1972). *Suicide and grief.* Philadelphia: Fortress Press.
Tatelbaum, J. (1980). *The courage to grieve.* New York: Harper and Row.
Veninga, R. (1985). *A gift of hope.* Boston: Little, Brown.
Westberg, G. (1961). *Good grief.* Philadelphia: Fortress Press.
Wrobleski, A. (1984). *Suicide: Your child has died.* Available from Adina Wrobleski, 5124 Grove Street, Minneapolis, MN 55436.

Homicide

Cairns, R. (1986, Spring). Predicting aggression in girls and boys. *Social Science, 71*(1), 16–21.
Coalter, F. (1985, January). Crowd behavior at football matches: A study in Scotland. *Leisure Studies, 4*(1), 111–117.
Collison, B. B., Bowden, S., Patterson, H., Snyder, J., et al. (1987, March). After the shooting stops [Special issue: Counseling and violence]. *Journal of Counseling and Development, 65*(7), 389–390.
Dominick, R. (1984, Spring). Videogames, television violence, and aggression in teenagers. *Journal of Communication, 34*(2), 136–1447.
Doyle, P. (1980). *Grief counseling and sudden death: A manual and guide.* Springfield, IL: Charles C. Thomas.
Dunham, R. G., & Alpert, G. P. (1987, Spring). Keeping juvenile delinquents in school: A prediction model. *Adolescence, 22*(85), 45–57.
Eastwood, L. (1985). Personality, intelligence and personal space

among violent and non-violent delinquents. *Personality and Individual Differences, 6*(6), 717-723.

Finckenauer, J. O., & Kochis, D. S. (1984). Causal theory and the treatment of juvenile offenders: A case study. *Advances in Forensic Psychology and Psychiatry, 1*, 49-63.

Huey, W. C., & Rank, R. C. (1984). Effects of counselor and peer-led group assertive training on black adolescent aggression. *Journal of Counseling Psychology, 31*(1), 95-98.

Jaffe, P., Wilson, S., & Wolfe, D. A. (1986, October). Promoting changes in attitudes and understanding of conflict resolution among child witnesses of family violence [special issue: Family violence: Child abuse, and wife assault]. *Canadian Journal of Behavioral Science, 18*(4), 356-366.

Kelly, J. A., St. Lawrence, J. S., Bradlyn, A. S., Himadi, W. G., Graves, K. A., & Keane, T. M. (1982, March). Interpersonal reactions to assertive and unassertive styles when handling social situations. *Journal of Behavioral Therapy and Experimental Psychiatry, 13*(1), 33-40.

Klepinger, D. H., & Weis, J. G. (1985, December). Projecting crime rates: An age, period, and cohort model using arima techniques. *Journal of Quantitative Criminology, 1*(4), 387-416.

Lefebvre-Pinard, M., & Reid, L. (1980, March). A comparison of three methods of training communication skills: Social conflict, modeling, and conflict-modeling. *Child Development, 51*(1), 179-187.

Lefer, L. (1984, April). The fine edge of violence. *Journal of the American Academy of Psychoanalysis, 12*(2), 253-268.

Leyva, F. A., & Furth, H. G. (1986, March). Compromise formation in social conflict: The influence of age, issue and interpersonal context. *Journal of Youth and Adolescence, 9*(1), 17-27.

Magie, D. (1983). *What murder leaves behind.* New York: Dodd, Mead.

May, J. M. (1986, March). Cognitive processes and violent behavior in young people. *Journal of Adolescence, 9*(1), 17-27.

Nagaraja, J. (1985). Psychodynamic of the acting-out belligerent youth. *Child Psychiatry Quarterly, 18*(4), 130-134.

Okeeffe, N. K., Brockopp, K., & Chew, E. (1986). Teen dating violence. *Social Work, 31*(6), 465-468.

Romney, D. M., & Syverson, K. L. (1984). An attempt to identify the personality dimensions of the violent offender. *Social Behavior and Personality, 12*(1), 53-60.

Roscoe, B., & Kelsey, T. (1986). Dating violence among high school students. *Psychology: A Quarterly Journal of Human Behavior, 23*(1), 53-59.

Sprafkin, J., & Gadow, K. B. (1986). Television viewing habits of emotionally disturbed, learning disabled, and mentally retarded children. *Journal of Applied Developmental Psychology, 7*(1), 45-59.

Vander Werff, J. J. (1985, December). Individual problems of self-definition: An overview, and a view. *International Journal of Behavioral Development, 8*(4), 445-71.

Van-De-Vliert, E. (1981, September). Siding and other reactions to a conflict: A theory of escalation toward outsiders. *Journal of Conflict Resolution, 25*(3), 495-520.

Weissberg, R. P., & Gesten, E. L. (1982, Winter). Considerations for developing effective school-based social problem-solving (SPS) training programs. *School Psychology Review, 11*(1), 56-63.

Younger, A. J., & Schwartzman, A. E. (1986, July). Age-related differences in children's perceptions of social deviance: Changes in behavior or in perspective? *Developmental Psychology, 22*(4), 531-542.

Sudden Death

Krupp, G. R., & Klegfield, B. (1962, November). Bereavement reactions: A cross cultural evaluation. *Journal of Religion and Health, 1*(3), 222-246.

Stickland, A. L., & DeSpelder, L. A. (1987). *The last dance: Encountering death and dying.* Palo Alto, CA: Mayfield.

Worden, J. W. (1982). Grief counseling and grief therapy. New York: Springer.

11

Chemical Dependency: The Adolescent and the Family

*William L. Harshman**

In crisis intervention we have learned that the presenting problem is frequently a defense against the real problem or threat facing the individual or family. The presentation of chemical dependency as a crisis is no different. Let's take a glance at some of the recent trends regarding adolescents and chemical consumption. According to Simpson 1989 the following are representative of today's youth:

1. 95% experiment with chemicals prior to their graduation from high school.
2. 70% of students grade 7–12 are current users (at least one time per month).
3. 90% of high school seniors have tried marijuana (1 out of 13 use it daily).

*This chapter has been excerpted and adapted by William Steele from the author's original unpublished article.

William Harshman, M.A., L.L.P., C.A.C., is a Certified Addiction Specialist whose expertise is in adolescent chemical dependency with emphasis on family involvement. He works with student assistance programs and has conducted numerous training programs for school personnel.

4. 40% of high school seniors display a history of poly-drug experimentation.
5. Approximately 30% of students grade 7-12 are using chemicals on a regular basis (at least one time per week).
6. Approximately 13% of students grade 7-12 are daily users.
7. Usage ratios between males and females have decreased in the past decade from 6:1 to 2:1.
8. The average age of first chemical use by males has decreased to 11.4 years.
9. The average age of first chemical use by females has decreased to 12.5 years.
10. The life expectancy is increasing for every age group except adolescents, who are dying at 15% greater rate than 20 years ago.
11. Suicides (at least 50% of which can be linked to the use of chemicals) take the lives of at least 35,000 adolescents per year, from an estimated 500,000 suicide attempts.
12. Males aged 16-19 are responsible for over 25% of all chemically related motor vehicle fatalities.
13. 50% of all serious crimes committed within the United States are committed by children aged 10-17. The crime rate of this population has increased 300% since 1960.
14. The average child watches over 20,000 hours of T.V. by the time he/she has reached high school graduation, including 360,000 commercials conveying the message that "Pain is unacceptable! You do not have to feel bad. . . . Medicate!"
15. 70% of all adolescents who display the characteristics of chemical dependency are children of at least one chemically dependent parent.

Additionally, Morrison and Talbott (in press) point out that one out of every five adolescents who abuse chemicals will cross the "genetic-wall' into full-blown chemical addiction.

In order to establish a comprehensive understanding as to the differences that exist between adolescent chemical use, abuse, and dependency, it is best to begin with what we know about the most pronounced condition, chemical dependency. There is an abundance of excellent resources on the treatment of chemical dependency. The success of any treatment or intervention, however, is dependent upon several critical factors. One of these factors is the identification and assessment of the real problem.

The following discussion makes us aware of some of the factors that must enter into any assessment of the role that chemicals play in an adolescent presenting what may appear to be a drug problem. This awareness is essential to an appropriate assessment of a crisis when substance abuse is presented as the major problem.

CAUTION WITH PROBLEM IDENTIFICATION

It is evident that the use, abuse, and experimentation of chemicals are taking a great toll on our adolescent population. We need to confront this issue, but we must do so with both caution and direction. Taking into consideration the diverse array of physiological, psychological, and sociological transitions experienced by an individual during adolescence, it is often simplistic and presumptuous on our part to conclude that chemical consumption is the *source* of any particular conflict. What I mean here is that adolescents by nature are going to experiment with extremes in both values and behavior. Fluctuating between periods of idealism and hedonism, adolescents are continually caught inside of the spiral of changes that occur in their ideals, behaviors, attitudes, and goals. As such, they are developmentally prone to great swings in mood and emotion, both of which affect behavior. All too often adults, caught up in the effects of this developmental spiral, seek a quick answer to the difficult question, "What is wrong with this child and what can be done to fix it?" And, all too often, if chemical use and/or experimentation is disclosed by the adolescent, then that becomes identified as the source of the conflict. When this occurs the child can be left unaided concerning the identification and resolution of developmental issues that may be altogether unrelated to the use of chemicals.

As Blum and Singer (1983) point out, most cases of adolescent deviance have multiple causative factors. Therefore, each case needs to be assessed in a differential diagnostic format that encompasses the totality of adolescent developmental issues. It is my belief, however, that chemical consumption by adolescents and its resultant effects are of major clinical importance.

THE FAMILY SYSTEM

Wegschieder (1980), Black (1982), Bradshaw (1988), and Forward and Buck (1989) all point to the necessity of incorporating the dysfunctional family system into an understanding of the disease of chemical dependency. Accepting the validity of a genetic predisposition, these studies have focused on the psycho-social effects of growing up within a dysfunctional family. They include not only chemically dependent families, but also families wherein chronic stress is evidenced through any of the folowing behaviors:

1. Incest/Sexual abuse
2. Physical abuse
3. Emotional abuse
4. Psychiatric illness
5. Compulsive gambling
6. Religious condemnation
7. Compulsive work activity
8. Compulsive eating disorders

Noting the prevalence of chronic stress within such families, these same authors have all suggested the identification of a "shame-based" family system that experientially suppresses the successful individuation of its members. Characterized by the three principles that Black (1982) refers to as (1) don't talk, (2) don't trust, and (3) don't feel, families such as these appear to produce children disproportionately prone to "addictive behavior." These children often experience and/or display one or more of the following psychological issues:

1. Low self-esteem
2. Poor self-concept
3. Impulsivity
4. Guilt
5. Shame
6. Fear
7. Emotional pain
8. Compulsivity
9. Poor reasoning ability

It therefore appears that children of dysfunctional, "shame-based" families present profiles wherein the root of their pathology can be traced to both genetic and intrapsychic origins. These are directly affected by the family system. Sociologically, the dysfunction of such a family tends to affect each member of the system both individually and collectively. The studies cited above also suggest that the dysfunctional family system becomes so enmeshed that it begins to normalize the dysfunction inherent to that system. As this occurs the family begins to adapt internally, often through a process of role-alteration, in the hope of maintaining the family system. In other words, the family as a group engages in self-defeating behaviors that reduce the threat they experience from the drinking and/or drug problems. They do not have the coping skills available to them that could actually resolve this crisis. Pervaded with extreme levels of denial, rationalization, and minimization, such families become invested in the maintenance of the very dysfunction that is creating the distress in the first place.

SOCIAL REINFORCEMENT

Considering this, Social Learning Theory proclaims that we tend to learn appropriate and/or dysfunctional mechanisms of social adaptation through our observations of persons of significance to us within our environmental setting. We then subsequently imitate that behavior (Bandura, 1969; Eysenck, 1970).

Suggesting that the imitation and maintenance of behavior is to a large degree contingent upon our experienced awareness and anticipation of the consequences of our actions, we tend to imitate behavior that evokes positive social reinforcement (Corsini & Marsello, 1983). As we have already seen, the chemically dependent family system, which is representative of the dysfunctional family system, appears to reinforce those behaviors that perpetuate its continuance. Individuals within such a setting are provided with a model of socialization that inhibits the construction of a personal identity that is based on appropriate mechanisms of social adaptation.

It must be remembered that the family system, to an extent, is representative of the environment in which it exists. As such, when considering those agents that affect social reinforcement, the following must be included:

1. Societal norms and customs
2. Ethnic norms and customs
3. Peer group norms and customs
4. Educational and institutional norms and customs
5. Religious and theological norms and customs
6. Media advertisement and promotion

When included in the construction of a developmental model of chemical dependency, it appears that these vehicles of socialization all have a pronounced influence upon the presence of chemical use within the family system. Royce (1981) cited that Americans spent $43.8 billion in 1979, or $120 million a day, on taxable alcoholic beverages alone! It seems reasonable to conclude that chemical use is a socially reinforced phenomenon within our culture. Further, it appears that those who are predisposed to the disease of chemical dependency within our society are pervaded with a multifactorial press towards chemical consumption that includes:

1. Physiological factors
2. Psychological factors
3. Sociological factors
4. Environmental factors

Therefore, because of both its genetic origin and the constant social reinforcement attached to this type of behavior, the disease of chemical dependency is, indisputably, a pervasive condition that cannot be addressed from a singular perspective.

ADOLESCENTS CARRYING ADULT SYMPTOMS

Continuing on this premise, these studies indicate that the socialization process, as a whole, has been altered in such a way that those developmental supports necessary for a stabilized maturation are, for the most part, no longer present within our society. It also appears that the developmental needs of our children are not being met, and as a result they are beginning to display increased levels of psychosocial pathology. According to Elkind (1981), adolescents who enter into the counseling milieu today are displaying the symptoms of stress usually associated with the adult population. Believing that these children have become overwhelmed by the pressures placed upon them by both their parents and society at large, he suggests that they are responding to these increased levels of stress through:

1. School failure
2. Delinquency
3. Alcohol/Drugs
4. Psychosomatic complaints
5. Apathy
6. Suicide

Confirming these findings, Morrison and Talbott (in press) and Blum and Singer (1983) also point out that when an adolescent experiences excessive stress and is not sophisticated enough to deal with it appropriately, he/she may begin to manifest it through:

1. Substance abuse
2. Sexual promiscuity

3. Criminal behavior
4. Social withdrawal
5. Hyperactivity
6. Truancy
7. Cult activity
8. Self-mutilation
9. Physical aggression

Considering this, it appears that children in our society are being rushed through their childhood in such a way that they are being deprived of the time and the opportunity to be children. As such, Elkind (1981) contends that adolescents are displaying not only increased levels of stress, but also the behavioral and psychological effects of its presence. To explain this phenomenon Elkind (1981, 1984) suggests that children no longer have the traditional family system at their disposal to assist them in their developmental struggles. And even if the family is intact the emphasis now appears to be placed on achievement, success, and competition. Due to the enormous social changes that have occurred during the past quarter of a century, he believes that our economy has been altered in ways that have directly impacted the structure of the family system. As a result, the roles that children play within the family have also been altered.

ADOLESCENTS PLAYING ADULT ROLES

According to Elkind (1981, 1984), the increases in both divorce and the need for dual-income households in this country are confronting children with issues that they were previously protected from. As such, many children are now left to fend for themselves while their parent(s) is/are out making a living. Because of this these children must not only deal with the demands of daily living, but also with the loneliness and sense of desertion that these types of situations can create. Additionally, he has suggested that parents often attempt to resolve their own feelings of guilt and shame for having placed their children in such a situation by pushing them towards success. Trying to prove to themselves and to the community in which they live that they are in fact "good parents," they pressure their children into academic and athletic achievement. Naturally, all of this pressure places great stress upon each member of the family.

ADOLESCENTS AS ADULTS' PARTNERS

Children within such a family often take on the role of "partner." Left in the home by themselves much of the time, they are called upon to make decisions that they are often not equipped to make. The added stress placed upon them by this demand not only taxes their limited decision-making skills, but additionally creates stresses for the child if such a decision does not work out. Elkind (1981, 1984) also claims that almost half of the children currently under the age of eighteen live in a single parent household. In addition to the stresses already addressed, these children are placed into an even more precarious situation. Not only must they deal with the reality that one of the parents is absent from the home but, they must also act as a support system for the parent with whom they reside. Elkind reminds us that the single parent is often separated from traditional avenues of support (spouse, friends, family) due to the fact that most of his or her time is spent either preparing for work or coming home from work. Because of this, it appears that single parents use their children as sounding boards upon which they can vent their frustrations. Here again, he reminds us that children placed in this situation have not developed the mental resources required to deal with adult issues, and any pressure placed upon them to do so, or to adapt to more mature levels of interaction, increases the stress they experience.

WHY CHEMICALS?

Adolescents are people too. And when confronted with a vast array of stressors of which they believe they have only limited control, they will seek out a means of lessening their stress. It is in this context that the experimentation with and use of chemicals by this population should be viewed. Pushed towards premature maturation, deprived of essential developmental support systems, and then saturated with media advertisements promoting their engagement in adult activities, it would seem odd if adolescents did not attempt to alleviate stress in much the same manner as does a large part of the adult population. Additionally, adolescents want to be wanted. And if that does not and/or is not possible within the confines of the family system, they will seek it out elsewhere. It is in this way that peer group affiliations have taken on such increased levels of significance for today's adolescent. Considering this, even those adolescents who reside within functional family systems are pressed towards conforming to their peer group's standards. Reiterating this process, Morrison and Talbott (in press) suggest that adolescents use chemicals to:

1. Have a good time.
2. Be a part of the group.
3. Get their minds off of their problems or escape.

WHEN IS IT "THE" PROBLEM?

It is not my belief that all adolescents who present a history of either chemical experimentation or use are displaying problematic behavior, in and of itself. However, the acknowledgment of such a history calls for further examination. Taking into consideration all of the predisposing factors confronting today's youth, and the disfranchisement of the traditional family system and its resultant effects upon the adolescent, the possible presence of a clinical diagnosis must be ruled out when chemical consumption and/or the correlate behaviors of such are identified! Considering this, those in contact with the adolescent population must be familiar not only with the issues regarding chemical dependency, but also with the other possible clinical manifestations of their behavior.

In determining the existence of a chemical dependency diagnosis it is imperative that the signs and symptoms representative of that diagnosis be identified. Failure to do so may result in the assignment of an improper diagnosis and the prescription of the wrong treatment (Beasley, 1987; Blum & Singer, 1983). It must be remembered that adolescents often display the characteristics of multiple issues. Therefore, caution must be taken in the identification and assignment of the primary diagnosis. As often occurs with adolescents displaying substance abuse histories but not chemical dependency diagnoses, their primary psychiatric issues have never been identified. As such, these issues continue to manifest themselves in such a way as to contaminate the improperly prescribed chemical dependency treatment regime.

ASSESSMENT

According to Jellinek (1960) there are 43 signs within the progressive pathology of chemical dependency. Naturally, an individual does not need to display all 43 before the diagnosis can be made, although it must be remembered that one sign does not a diagnosis make. It is my belief that there are five hallmark signs of the disease of chemical dependency. If at least four of these are present it is pretty much assured that many of Jellinek's signs will be found among them, and that the diagnosis can safely be made. These five signs are:

1. **Genetic predisposition.** The identification of at least one biological family member, within two generations, who displays a profile depicting chemical dependency.
2. **Increased tolerance/initial high tolerance.** A history of chemical use that indicates either the need for greater amounts of the chemical in order to produce the desired effect, or a limited chemical use history that includes the ability to consume great amounts of the chemical.
3. **Blackouts.** Chemically induced amnesia. The loss of memory following periods of intoxication.

4. **Loss of control.** The inability to predict one's behavior prior to the ingestion of the chemical.

5. **Continued use of the chemical, despite negative consequences.** A historical profile that includes physical, social, legal, and/or occupational problems that are the direct result of chemical use.

As was indicated earlier in this presentation, the assessment of an adolescent cannot be limited only to the individual and/ or the clinical issues that are directly related to the chemical consumption (Blum & Singer, 1983). Additionally, it must include the examination of:

1. Family status
2. Educational status
3. Vocational status
4. Physiological status
5. Psychological status
6. Social status
7. Legal status
8. Sexual status (including sexual abuse, incest, orientation, promiscuity, birth control, etc.)

Only through the inclusion of these variables is it possible to assess the holistic needs of the adolescent, and then determine the level of care needed to address the identified issues. For this reason the individual conducting the assessment needs to be not only prepared to investigate these issues, but also comfortable with the process. Naturally this includes an acknowledging of one's own limitations and a willingness to seek assistance with regard to areas beyond one's expertise.

SCHOOL SETTING

Many schools provide support groups for young people who have received outside intervention for their chemical problems and/or the chemical problems of their parents. These groups can indeed be very beneficial. Schools have now identified providing such support as a role appropriate to their setting, responsibilities, and capabilities. Is this role, however, one of assessment, and, if so, what is the extent of their assessment and what ought to be its purpose? It has been stated several times in previous chapters that the school setting is not a clinical setting and therefore is not the place to make a diagnosis and/or provide clinical treatment. School counselors should, however, be prepared to identify young people who are "at risk," and be able to assess both the seriousness of the situation and the immediate needs of a youth and his/her family, so as to provide the best possible intervention with the intent of preventing more serious crises from arising.

The goal of a school assessment when chemical usage is part of the presenting problem is to: (1) identify other possible core problems that may be marked by the chemical presentation; and (2) provide and encourage further outside examination so as to arrive at a clinical diagnosis of the youth's situation. Is the chemical presentation a chemical dependency problem or a manifestation of another diagnosis? This is a question that schools should not be expected to answer. Schools are expected to assess the potential dangers of a youth presenting a chemical problem, refer that youth to outside sources for a qualified diagnosis, and then, if they choose (and many do), provide the kind of support to the youth and his/her family that supports the healing and recovery process while complementing any therapeutic intervention that is being provided by outside resources.

FAMILY ASSESSMENT

Intervening with a family presenting a chemical crisis is no different than intervening with families presenting other crises. The stages remain the same, as do the questions related to the nature of the crisis and the kind of family system being utilized. The questions related to the actual use of the identified chemical will of course be different from questions that might be asked about a suicide crisis. A crisis team, or an individual assigned to providing crisis intervention, may or may not have specific knowledge related to the presenting problem. This does not have to reduce the effectiveness of the intervenor or the value of the initial assessment he/she can provide, however, since the focus of crisis intervention is assessing immediate danger and taking the action necessary to remove that danger as quickly as possible.

INTERVENTION

Even if an intervenor has little knowledge about chemical usage, he/she can, using the questions identified in the various stages, still determine a great deal about the potential risk levels of the family, the identified "problem member," the crisis, the strengths of the family system, its weaknesses, and the extent of its coping skills, problem-solving skills, and needs. With this information all of the parties can best determine how the school can help the family to come to a healthy resolution of this crisis. The stages of intervention remain the same. An intervenor who knows nothing about chemical dependency, but who followed the stages outlined in the previous chapters would: (1) know a great deal more after the intervention; (2) still be effective in helping the family understand their crisis differently; (3) be seen by the family as knowledgeable and supportive; (4) be able to provide problem-solving resolutions; and (5) help to reduce the tremendous anxiety accompanying their crisis, thereby allowing the family to take the action needed to restabilize, or return to their level of functioning prior to the crisis, or to become stronger as a family as a result of their acceptance of the intervention being provided.

RED FLAGS

"Don't talk, trust, or feel" were identified earlier as characterizing the "shame-based" family system. If you recall, they are also the characteristics seen in a closed family system. In the "shame-based" family these factors tend to be very prevalent. Denial, rationalization, and the minimization of problems are also characteristic of these two systems, which for our purposes are one and the same. The more prevalent these factors are, the higher the risk and the greater the need for clinical intervention. Resolution also becomes more difficult to achieve when these factors exist.

The discussion of closed family systems in stage four of Chapter 7 and shown in Table 2.1 reflect the "shame-based" family characteristics listed below:

"Don't talk." The closed family system is secretive and has a restrictive communication pattern.

"Don't trust." and "Don't feel." Affection (feeling) is very covert in closed families, and the emotional bonds are built more on fear than on trust.

As you review the information about closed families you'll remember that this system's focus is to maintain a family image of unity despite the chaos and conflict that frequently exist in families where chemical dependency exists. The "enabling behavior" that exists in these families is very much directed toward concealing from those outside of the family the real problems that exist, problems that the family members themselves are ashamed of.

This does not suggest that change is not possible, but only that it may be more difficult to achieve, as chemical abuse clinicians know all too well. From a school's perspective, however, the opportunity does exist to be helpful to students of such a family by increasing their understanding of the workings of their family (a different cognitive understanding of the crisis), and of the ways (problem solve) they can care for themselves despite the conditions that exist. Keep in mind that such a family system in crisis is vulnerable, and that during this vulnerability they will be, to some degree, open to managing their crisis differently, although still within the framework of their system.

REFERENCES

Beasley, J. D. (1987). *Wrong diagnosis–wrong treatment: The plight of the alcoholic in America.* New York: Creative Infomatics.

Bandura, A. (1969) *Principles of behavior modification.* New York: Holt, Rinehart and Winston.

Black, C. (1982). *It will never happen to me.* Denver, CO: MAC Book Department.

Blum, K., & Singer, E. P. (Eds.). (1983). The psychobiology of alcoholism [Special issue]. *Substance and Alcohol Actions/ Misuse 4.*

Bradshaw, J. (1988). *Healing the shame that binds you.* Hollywood, FL: Health Communications.

Corsini, R., & Marsello, A. (1983). *Personality theories, research and assessment.* Itasca, IL: F. E. Peacock.

Elkind, D. (1981). *The hurried child: Growing up too fast too soon.* Reading, MA: Addison-Wesley.

Elkind, D. (1984). *All grown up and no place to go.* Reading, MA: Addison-Wesley.

Eysenck, H. J. (1970). *The structure of human personality* (3rd ed.). London: Methuen.

Forward, S., & Buck, C. (1989). *Toxic parents: Overcoming their hurtful legacy and reclaiming your life.* New York: Bantam.

Jellinek, E. M. (1960). *The disease concept of alcoholism.* Highland Park, NJ: Hillhouse Press.

Morrison, M., & Talbott, G. (in press). Adolescence and vulnerability to chemical dependence. In *Adolescent substance abuse and dependence* (booklet). (Available from Talbott Recovery Systems, 1669 Phoenix Parkway, Suite 102, Atlanta, GA 30349.)

Royce, J. E. (1981). *Alcohol problems and alcoholism: A comprehensive study.* New York: Free Press.

Simpson, D. (1989, September 20). Adolescent chemical dependency: Making lives count. *Professional Education Series.* Albion, MI: Starr Commonwealth School.

Wegschieder, S. (1980). *Another chance: Hope and help for the alcoholic family.* Palo Alto, CA: Science and Behavior Books.

12

Crisis Intervention with Sexual Minority Youth and Their Families: An Overview for Educators

Michael W. Hazelton*

DISCOVERY

I tried to kill myself when I was 11 years old. I think I even sort of knew at that age that I didn't fit into the world at all. Then, I tried to tell my parents that I was a lesbian when I was 15. They told me that they were going to send me back to the psychiatrist. Now, one of my greatest fears is that they will disown me.

Heather,** now 27 years old, is preparing, once again, to tell her parents that she is a lesbian.

*Michael W. Hazelton, M.S.W., is a psychiatric social worker who has broad experience with sexual issues, particularly as they relate to suicide in gay and lesbian adolescents and young adults.

**Personal discussions with Heather, David, Kevin, Kirk, Jeff, a high school counselor, and a middle-aged gay man were conducted between January 1989 and August 1990. All identifying information has been altered to protect confidentiality. The discussions yielded a wealth of information. Unfortunately, it is beyond the scope of this chapter to include more of the discussion content. The author wishes to express his deepest gratitude to the participants for their openness and candor.

David recalls his parents' response when he told them that he was gay.

> When I came out to them it was kind of [peculiar]. My father just sort of focused on one object in my living room. You could definitely tell he was in shock. My mother just started firing questions. It was like I was standing in front of a firing squad and her questions were bullets. They just came one right after the other.

Kirk remembers that his mother "freaked like everybody probably does" when he told her he was gay. "She got all flushed and asked me if I was afraid of girls or something. Then she told me that she always knew I was different. My parents were O.K. with it at first. Within about a year they became very positive and supportive."

One of the most devastating crises that a family can face is the discovery that a child is lesbian, gay, bisexual, or transsexual. Even in highly functional families where communication is open, rules and roles are flexible, and external support systems are available, the nonheterosexual orientation of a member can serve to undermine the family's normal abilities to solve crises. DeVine (1984) has postulated that this discovery

> becomes a major crisis for the family system because: (1) there are no rules in the family system appropriate to handle the behavior, (2) there are no roles in the family specific to the issue into which the family members can fit, (3) there is no constructive language available to describe the issue, (4) there are strong negative family and cultural proscriptions against homosexual behavior, [and] (5) the cohesive element, regulative structure and themes within the family system become critical forces against adaptation. (p. 9)

Societal taboos, irrational fears, and the often deeply rooted hatred of homosexuality may make reliance on the usual external supports too threatening for the family. Self-blame by parents ("Where did we go wrong?"), and fear among siblings of being identified as gay or lesbian themselves if they discuss the issue with others, may cause the family to become isolated. Shrouded in guilt, afraid of discovery by friends and associates, and lacking the proper information, the families of sexual minorities often choose to avoid or deny the revelation altogether. Thus, in an effort to restore equilibrium and stability, even a family system that is normally open may suddenly become closed and rigid. Lacking the appropriate rules and roles, as well as the language that could help the family to adapt, the system rapidly becomes disorganized, boundaries become blurred, and the members may begin to perceive the family to be a failure.

Frequently the family responds by trying to remove the stressor, the homosexual child, from the system (DeVine, 1984). This can be accomplished through either emotional distancing or physical removal. Gay and lesbian young people are often either forced to leave home or they choose to run away from what has become an unbearable situation. They are also at high risk of attempting suicide after their rejection, or perceived rejection, by their families. Those from abusive and dysfunctional families are at an even higher risk (Gibson, 1989).

WHAT IS A SEXUAL MINORITY?

For the purposes of this chapter, sexual minorities include homosexual, bisexual, and transsexual people. The terms "gay," "lesbian," "homosexual," and "sexual minority" are used interchangeably. The author does not intend to minimize the special concerns of any particular group. However, detailed discussions of these specific concerns are beyond the scope of this report. Therefore, the focus of this chapter is to discuss the issues that affect all sexual minorities.*

*The author recommends reading additional material regarding the specific concerns of various sexual minority populations (see *References* and *Additional Reading* sections of this chapter). The intent of this chapter is to present an overview of sexual minority concerns and an introduction to appropriate crisis intervention with this population and their families.

RELEVANCE TO SCHOOLS

Many adults, including a number of educators and parents, believe that discussions of sex and sexuality have no place in the schools, and should be dealt with exclusively at home by parents. For whatever reasons, there is a tendency to deny both that young people are sexual beings and, based upon some serious misconceptions, that homosexuality simply does not exist among the young. A high school counselor reports:

> I was approached by a 16-year-old who told me he was gay and wanted my advice because his family refused to talk to him since the time he told them. Having no idea what to tell him, I went to the vice-principal who told me that homosexuality is not an appropriate issue for the school to deal with since it is too controversial, and we never encounter it in our district. As a result, I told the kid that I would refer him to a therapist so he could sort out his sexual confusion. Two days later he was back in my office reporting suicidal feelings. At that point, I realized that I had completely missed the boat.

In their landmark study, Bell, Weinberg, and Hammersmith (1981) report that there is strong evidence that sexual orientation is predisposed from an early age and may well have a biological foundation. In other words, young gay and lesbian people exist. Whether or not they are identified as such is another matter. David, now 30 years old, recalls that "in retrospect, and now that I have come to grips with my sexuality, I can realize back as far as 4 years old having dreams which were very sexually arousing and they always had to do with other [males]. It wasn't until near the end of my graduate studies that I saw not telling my family as a roadblock to getting on with my life".

Based upon accepted studies (Kinsey, Pomeroy, & Martin, 1948; Kinsey, Pomeroy, Martin, & Gebhard, 1953; Bell, Weinberg, and Hammersmith, 1981) we can estimate that in any school about one in ten students is destined to be predominantly homosexual. Using this 10% estimate, Griffin, Wirth, and Wirth (1986) calculate that there are some 24 million gay and lesbian people in the United States, 8 million of whom are under 18 years of age. Considering that these young people have parents and siblings, over 30 million family members are affected by the homosexual orientation of people under the age of 18. In fact, disregarding age, it is estimated that homosexuals and their parents constitute about one third of the population (Woodman, 1985). Therefore, the probability is very high that a teacher, counselor, or school administrator will encounter students and family members experiencing crises related to sexual orientation. "From nursery school through college, the teacher is the one professional who is sure to have contact with every developing Gay person" (Clark, 1987, p. 222).

Contrary to what many people would like to believe, the statistics regarding sexuality and sexual activity among young people are significant. The average age of the onset of intercourse is 16.2 years for females and 15.7 years for males (Zelnick & Shah, 1983), and each year one in seven teenagers is diagnosed with a sexually transmitted disease (House Select Committee on Children, Youth, and Families, 1987). Therefore, regardless of any intense societal denial, it is clear that many young people of all sexual orientations are exploring sexuality and are sexually active.

Sexual activity, suicide, homicide, child abuse, substance abuse, and numerous other issues affect contemporary families and schools. The families of young gays and lesbians are certainly no exceptions. In fact, they are at a much higher risk of experiencing problems such as suicide and violence. Consider the following facts:

- Suicide is the leading cause of death among sexual minority youth in the United States (Gibson, 1989). It is the third leading cause among the same age group in the general population (Centers for Disease Control, 1985).
- Sexual minority youth are two to three times more likely to attempt suicide than other young people (Gibson, 1989).
- Gay and lesbian youth comprise up to 30% of all completed youth suicides annually (Gibson, 1989). This is

particularly alarming since they comprise only about 10% of the total youth population.

- The majority of all suicide attempts made by homosexual individuals occur at or before the age of twenty, with almost one third of those occurring before the age of seventeen (Bell & Weinberg, 1978).
- Sexual minorities are frequently the targets of verbal and physical assaults because of their sexual orientation, indicating premeditation on the part of assailants (Bohn, 1983).
- In over 93% of the cases of harassment and assault, gay and lesbian victims report that they do not know their assailants (Bohn, 1983). Whereas, in the general population three out of five victims know their assailants (Federal Bureau of Investigation, 1986). In other words, sexual minorities are much more likely to be victims of random violence.
- The root problem of sexual minority youth suicide [and victimization] is social stigmatization and discrimination (Gibson, 1989).

In many situations the school environment itself serves to place gay and lesbian youth at risk. Rarely is homosexuality addressed in the curricula, and there is little or no access to positive information about the subject in school settings. Students who are suspected of being homosexuals are ridiculed, isolated, and often physically attacked by peers. Teachers are afraid to intervene in the harassment of gay and lesbian students for fear of being regarded as undesirable role models (Parris, 1985), or of being identified as gay themselves (Tartagni, 1978). Students who hide their homosexual identity often choose to isolate themselves to keep from being discovered. Heather recalls her junior and senior high school experiences:

[I]t was very popular to walk into school and hear kids bashing gays and lesbians. Usually they didn't use those words though. You'd hear [words] like "fag," "dyke," or "queer." It was like an obsession [for them]. [One day] this guy in the hall kicked me and almost destroyed one of my eyes. He thought it was very funny that he had "almost blinded a queer," and he bragged to his friends about it. Most of the time the teachers would just sit back and pretend they didn't see anything. Maybe they were scared to get involved.

Donna Tartagni, a high school counselor, believes that "the loneliest person in the country is the gay in the typical high school of today" (Norton, 1976, p. 376). It is common knowledge among suicide experts that social isolation is a critical risk factor in youth suicide. From this perspective, schools must take on the crucial responsibility for providing appropriate crisis intervention, and for creating the environmental changes necessary to reduce the disproportionate risks faced by sexual minority youth and their families. The first step toward achieving this is to correct some of the most prevalent misconceptions about homosexuality.

COMMON MISCONCEPTIONS

Teachers, counselors, and other professionals often claim that they have never encountered a young gay or lesbian person ("We don't have that problem in our school, program, culture, etc."). Most often, this belief actually reflects the fact that they have not encountered a young person who has openly and assertively identified him- or herself as gay or lesbian. When asked what they would do if they did encounter such a person, some report that they would attempt to help the person to "change to a healthier lifestyle." Others have no idea what they would do. Though well intended, these responses are based upon serious misconceptions about sex, sexuality, and sexual orientation. A discussion of several of the more common misconceptions follows.

Misconception: People Choose the Homosexual "Lifestyle"

A middle-aged gay man reported that a young lesbian friend once asked, "Why do we choose to be homosexuals?" He

replied, "No one in their right mind would choose to be gay
or lesbian in this world! It's just the way we are." She retorted,
"I chose my lifestyle!" This is a classic example of how the
concepts of sexual orientation and "lifestyle" are often confused. Gay and lesbian people come from every walk of life,
culture, race, creed, economic class, political party, and lifestyle. To assume that homosexuality is a lifestyle is to assume
that all homosexuals fit a certain stereotyped image. In addition, those who do fit the stereotype are often subjected to
abuse. Heather attributes a great deal of the abuse she suffered
in school to the fact that "I sort of fit the stereotype. So, I was
an easy target for people that were just sort of insecure about
who they were. By not fitting into the typical 'girl' role, I
brought out feelings of hostility in people."

As previously noted, it is well documented that sexual
orientation is formed before adolescence, and that there is
strong evidence of a biological basis for its development.
Pomeroy (1972), who worked with Dr. Alfred Kinsey on pio-
neer studies of sexuality, recalls the surprise of the researchers
at finding that homosexuality occurs as often in other species
as it does in humans. The author whimsically recounts a
statement made by an eminent sex researcher, who after reviewing a film that confirmed homosexual activity among
other species, quipped: "Every judge in the country who has
to deal with sex offenders should see this film. It might teach
him [or her] something about what the word 'unnatural'
means"* (p. 183). Lifestyles are chosen, sexual orientation is
not; it occurs naturally.

Griffin, Wirth, and Wirth (1986) point out that the concepts of choice and change are closely interrelated in the
public mind. In other words, "if someone chooses to be gay,
he or she can choose not to be gay" (p. 34). As an experiment,
try to imagine what would happen if you asked a "known"
heterosexual why he or she chose to be "straight." Chances
are you would receive a very strange look, and perhaps even a

*The use of the term "sex offenders" by the researcher was clearly in
reference to those who are arrested for homosexual activity and was not
intended to refer to those guilty of sexual assault, molestation, etc.

punch in the mouth. If you are feeling really testy, imagine what would happen if you suggested that this person should seek professional help in order to change his or her sexual orientation. This person would probably suggest that you are the one who needs some help. For most heterosexual-oriented people there is never any question of choice. They are never faced with "admitting" their orientation, nor are they described as "practicing" heterosexuals. After all, why on earth would anyone have to "practice" that which comes naturally? More importantly, how can anyone be expected to change an innate characteristic? It is no different for nonheterosexual people.

Sexual minority youth are burdened with rejection and disdain for who they are. Suggestions that they should change themselves convey the message that they are somehow bad people. Sexuality and sexual orientation are integral elements at the core of the personality, and so it is essential to discard the notion that sexual orientation is a choice that can be changed. Otherwise, one out of ten children will face a very bleak future.

Misconception: Homosexuality Is Contagious

One of the greatest injustices suffered by gay and lesbian people is the denial of basic human rights. News publications are replete with stories about gay teachers being fired, convicted murderers being given light sentences because the victims were homosexuals, denial of adoption and foster care rights to gay and lesbian couples, evictions of people suspected of having AIDS, and scandals about "suspected" homosexual political and religious leaders. Adult homosexuals who associate with young people are suspected of, if not criminally charged with, attempting to "recruit" or "seduce" children into homosexuality. Heterosexual professionals often fear associating with homosexual colleagues because they may be suspected of being gay or lesbian themselves. These kinds of responses to homosexuality suggest an underlying fear of contagion.

The truth is that, as Bell, Weinberg, and Hammersmith (1981) found, there is a significant period of time between becoming aware of a homosexual orientation and acting upon it. The authors learned that neither gays nor lesbians were "seduced" or "recruited" into homosexuality. Kevin illustrates this point.

> I was probably 13 [years old] or so when I realized that I found men erotic and not women. But amazingly enough, I didn't act on these feelings until I was 20 or so. I didn't even go to a gay bar or have any gay friends until I was 28. I [had] moved my sexual identity to the "back forty" on the Ponderosa.

The belief that gay men tend to be child molesters (recruiters) was dispelled by research presented at the Fourth National Conference on Child Abuse and Neglect (Star, 1979). This confirmed that most of all child molestation is perpetrated by adult heterosexual males. In addition, Bohn (1984) found that of all reported male rapes, "most are committed by heterosexual men against gay men or youth," and represent the "ultimate expression of negating the [gay male's] masculinity" (p. 94).

The concept of contagion encourages the isolation of sexual minorities, not only from the general population but also from each other. Gay and lesbian youth, each of whom may already fear that he or she is the "only one," are prevented from discovering adults who could become positive gay role models. In schools, out of a fear of causing young people to become homosexuals, social activities for sexual minority students are prohibited, the contributions of gay and lesbian historical figures are not studied, and students are not taught that homosexuality occurs naturally within the continuum of sexual orientation. Public response to the AIDS crisis has served to promote the idea that homosexual activity equals death. Rather than admitting that young people are sexual beings and teaching them realistic ways to protect themselves, lawmakers have chosen to require school officials to teach abstinence, especially from same-sex activities. As a result, sexual minority youth are made to believe that the only responsible sex is no sex, ever. AIDS is contagious and preventable, and everyone who is sexually active is at risk. Homosexuality is neither contagious nor preventable, and no one can catch it.

Misconception: Homosexuality Is an Illness

There is no significant difference between the mental health of homosexuals and heterosexuals (Hooker, 1957). Neither the American Psychiatric Association nor the American Psychological Association regard homosexuality as a mental illness. In fact, researchers have found that, given the overwhelming odds and the degree of adversity faced by lesbians and gay men, not only are the majority of them psychologically healthy (Gonsiorek, 1982), but some may actually be healthier, in an overall sense, than heterosexuals (Freedman, 1975).

The "illness" concept is related to the psychoanalytic premise that homosexuality can be "cured." However, based upon his extensive experience in treating gay men, Isay (1989) suggests that traditional psychoanalytic theory, which asserts that homosexuality is the result of disruptions in normal development caused by early conflict, is actually derived "from social prejudice, which, in this instance, causes social values to be confused with health values" (p. 4). It is interesting to note that even the "Father of Psychoanalytic Theory," Freud (1903), directly stated that "homosexuals are not sick," and that they "must not be treated as sick people" (p. 5).

Psychoanalytic theory also suggests that either gender identity disturbances or arrested development can cause homosexuality, and therefore this "condition" can also be cured with the proper treatment. In the first place, gender identity and sexual orientation are related, yet discrete components of the whole person. Gender identity refers to the identification of oneself as male or female. Most adolescents engage in nonconforming behavior (e.g., unusual hair styles, males wearing earrings, etc.), and although gender nonconformity is common among gay youth, it is more likely a means of affirming their identity and not a cause of homosexual orientation (Gibson, 1989). On the other hand, sexual orientation has to do with one's affectional preference or sexual attraction to others. In other words, gay men do not perceive themselves as women trapped in male bodies, nor do lesbians desire to grow male genitalia. Lesbians are women, who are attracted to women, and gay men are men, who are attracted to men. Bisexuals are attracted to both sexes.

Though some young homosexuals may appear to be developmentally immature (arrested development), this is most often the result of their being deprived of opportunities to complete normal developmental tasks. Sexual minority youths lack positive role models, peer support, and the social sanctions usually needed to explore and develop intimate relationships. Normal development cannot occur in isolation. Arrested development does not cause homosexuality. The response of others to homosexuality causes arrested development.

To illustrate just how deeply ingrained such misconceptions can be, a professor at a major graduate school of social work included these two questions on a final exam in a clinical practice course:

What are the known causes of heterosexuality?
What are the known cures of heterosexuality?

Only a few students got the point. The rest stood in line, waiting patiently to point out the typographical errors to the professor.

"'Curing' homosexuals is as unlikely as 'curing' heterosexuals of their attraction to the [opposite] sex" (Cook, 1988, p. 7). It is a common mistake to assume that the homosexual orientation of the young person seeking help is *the problem*. This assumption runs contrary to the principles of crisis intervention. In all probability, *the problem* for the young lesbian or gay person who is seeking help is the way in which others have responded to her or his sexual orientation. In Chapter 8, Steele and Raider refer to these kinds of assumptions as "different cognitive understandings" of the problem. Heather recalls, "I never told my parents because [one of] my greatest fears was being subjected to forced psychiatric treatment." From this perspective, it is important for those who deal with sexual minority youth and their families in times of crisis, to be able to clarify the problem without becoming a part of the problem.

Misconception: Homosexual Behavior
Is Just a Phase

All adolescents go through "phases." Given the rapid physical, emotional, intellectual, and sexual changes they must endure, it's a wonder that anyone survives this period of life. Adolescents must also accomplish some formidable tasks, such as developing a sense of autonomy, establishing a positive identity, developing peer and intimate relationships, and acquiring a sense of the future. In order to do so, and with virtually no experience, they will test limits and rebel against that which is familiar, all in an effort to establish a sense of independence.

Gay and lesbian adolescents are no different in this regard. However, they face these challenges without the same support and tolerance afforded their nonhomosexual peers. Jeff, a 17-year-old, gay student at a suburban high school, illustrates this point:

> I consider myself to be very athletic, but I hate participating in school sports and gym class. Being in the locker room is the worst! All these guys stand around naked discussing who got laid, how many times, and what they're gonna do to score with this or that girl. If they knew what I was feeling, they would kill me. As a matter of fact, one guy, who I always thought was gay, got nailed by some of these guys when a gay newspaper fell out of his gym bag. Within an hour, the word was out all over school that he was a faggot. After school that day, a bunch of guys cornered him and beat him up pretty bad. I don't know what ever happened to him. I heard that he dropped out of school and went to live with his older brother in some other town.
>
> It's really hard seeing something like that, ya know? I really want to be able to talk to other kids about things that are important to me. But I'm just too scared. I guess I'll just have to wait until I'm out of here to make real friends. That really sucks!

Gay and lesbian youth often report feeling invisible and alone. If they are open about who they are, they face ridicule, rejection, and possibly physical abuse. If they keep their true identity a secret, they must live a lie and pass as "straight" (Gibson, 1989). Either way, they face huge obstacles to their accomplishing of normal developmental tasks. To confuse homosexual orientation with rebellious behavior or a phase is to deprive the adolescent of the opportunity to achieve a positive sense of self. When working with the families of sexual minority youth it is imperative to help them make this distinction. Even if the family is able to accept the homosexual orientation of their child, they will still have to cope with the normal adolescent "phases."

Misconception: Homosexuals Are Anti-family

In the preface to *Homosexuality and the Family,* Bozett (1989) quotes from a 1980 sermon in which a well-known evangelist minister flatly declared that "Homosexuals are anti-family." In late 1989, the U.S. Secretary of Health and Human Services capitulated to the demands of two legislators and repudiated sections of a federal report on youth suicide that document a significantly higher rate of suicide among sexual minority youth than among other youth. The sections of the *Report of the Secretary's Task Force on Youth Suicide* (Alcohol, Drug Abuse, and Mental Health Administration, 1989) were denounced on the basis that they "failed to affirm traditional family values" (Zeh, 1989).

Declarations such as these by civic and religious leaders are common in today's society. Strommen (1990) writes, "It is common knowledge that homosexuality is the subject of continuing and long standing hostility on the part of the majority of Americans" (p. 11). The author also points out that there is a widespread misconception that homosexuality constitutes a threat to children (Martin & Hetrick, 1988). Since children are the core focus of families, any perceived threat to the children is considered to pose a real and serious danger to the entire family. As a result, homosexuals are often denied positive relationships with children.

The belief that homosexuals are dangerous to the institution of the family is perhaps the most deeply rooted misconception of all. It is based solely upon social prejudice. This type of bias persists despite well-documented evidence that it is false (Burgess, et al., 1978; DeFrancis, 1966; Groth & Birnbaum, 1978; Kempe & Kempe, 1984). The word "prejudice" is defined as an "Irrational hatred of a particular group, race, or religion" (Davies, 1980, p. 556). People tend to hate that which they fear, and irrational hatred is based upon irrational fears, or phobias. The term used to describe this irrational fear of homosexuals is "homophobia."

Phobias are considered to be neurotic disorders by the American Psychiatric Association (1987), and neuroses are described as pathological, or ill, behavior patterns. It is sadly ironic that homosexuality is denounced as an evil sickness, despite strong evidence to the contrary, by those who promote themselves as the "healthiest of the healthy," and also despite all of the evidence to the contrary. Perhaps the saying "those who scream the loudest have the most to hide" bears some truth.

This is not to suggest that everyone who has misconceptions or fears about homosexuality is mentally ill. Rather, the intention is to expose the root problem faced by sexual minorities and their families. No one, regardless of sexual orientation, is exempt from homophobia. In fact, many gay and lesbian people who seek psychotherapy for feelings of guilt, self-hatred, and depression, are actually suffering from the effects of internalized homophobia (Malyon, 1982). Homophobia is also responsible for the victimization of and for suicides among sexual minority youth. As Gibson (1989) states, "The homophobia experienced by gay youth in all parts of their lives is the primary reason for their suicidal feelings" (p. 133).

Assertions that homosexuals are "anti-family" are patently irrational, or homophobic. Homosexual people are both products and members of families. Most of them cherish their families and the values that their families hold. Those who are forced to leave their families because of their homosexual orientation experience profound, long lasting grief. David and Heather both recalled fearing that their families would literally disown them upon learning of their sexual orientation. Thus, they kept their secrets well into adulthood.

It is heterosexual activity that produces homosexual children in the first place, and in almost all cases it is heterosexual parents who rear homosexual children. This in no way means that parents are to be "blamed" for their children's homosexuality. Bell, Weinberg, and Hammersmith (1981) provide comforting advice:

> [P]eople who criticize the parents of homosexuals for what they view as an aberration will have no cause to lay blame on them, while parents of gays may be relieved of whatever guilt they have felt about their parenting. There is a growing consensus, to which our own data lend support, that not much can be predicted about an individual on the basis of his or her parental relationships. (p. 219)

Ideally, the family provides a safe place where its members are cared for, protected, and nurtured with unconditional love. However, homophobia can be powerfully destructive to the families of lesbians and gays. As noted in the first section of this chapter, guilt, self-blame, and a lack of information and/or external supports can plunge even the most functional family into complete disarray upon the discovery that a member is gay or lesbian. For religious families the results can be catastrophic. As Strommen (1990) observes,

> Outdated interpretation and inappropriate use of scripture to justify the persecution of homosexuals has a long tradition in Christian society (Boswell, 1980; McNeill, 1988; Martin, 1984). While a minority of churches challenge anti-homosexual theology, the vast majority of Jewish and Christian faiths maintain a hostile attitude toward homosexuals in their flock (Hiltner, 1980). This doctrinal hostility means that families with strong religious convictions are likely to endorse this hostility, even against one of their own. (p. 12)

When dealing with the families of sexual minorities it is crucial to address homophobia through proper education and support. This means that teachers, counselors, and administrators must confront their own fears and misconceptions, and must educate themselves with rationality. They must commit themselves to creating an environment where sexual minorities are protected from abuse, afforded opportunities to achieve the normal tasks of adolescence, and supported in their personal growth. When providing crisis intervention to the families of sexual minorities it is essential to try to prevent the disintegration of the family structure whenever possible. It is only through this approach that "traditional family values" can be protected and maintained.

Misconception: Homosexuals Should Keep Their Sexual Orientation to Themselves

Many people wonder why gays and lesbians make such a big deal about revealing their sexual orientation. After all, heterosexuals don't feel compelled to announce their hetero-sexual orientation. Therein lies the difference. Most people tend to assume that everyone is heterosexual until told other-wise. For the homosexual person this assumption leaves only two choices. They must either hide or reveal a major aspect of their lives. David chose to keep his secret for many years:

> [My homosexuality] was a secret that I was going to keep forever. I was never going to tell anyone and I was going to end up married to a woman. [Now] I regret having kept it a secret for all those years. It was a period of no emotional growth. I became very effective at denying, burying, and hiding my feelings. So much so that, when I started to get back in touch with them, it was very hard for me to let them surface. I was just a whiz at that. It was bad news.

Sometimes people decide to "come out" so that others don't unexpectedly find out. "When parents or friends of lesbians and gays inadvertently discover a loved one's homosexuality they are often hurt or disappointed that they were not taken into confidence" (Schneider, 1988, p. 97). In addition, when it is discovered inadvertently an individual can be caught off guard, with no time to prepare for the disclosure. She or he may then face a crisis of major proportions. There is also evidence that suggests that those who stay in the "closet" are more likely than those who "come out" to have negative feelings about being gay (Lee, 1977; McDonald, 1982).

In *Often Invisible: Counselling Gay and Lesbian Youth,*
Margaret Schneider (1988) points out that although there are
risks involved for those who choose to come out, "self-disclo-
sure alleviates stress and its accompanying symptoms, pro-
motes a sense of identity, and contributes to higher self-
esteem" (p. 98). On the other hand, as Gibson (1989) points
out, gay and lesbian youth who are open about their sexual
orientation "remain at high risk to suicidal feelings and
behavior because of the pressures they face in conflicts with
others about their homosexual orientation" (p. 121). Making
the choice of whether or not to come out is often very difficult. For lesbian and gay youth seeking assistance with such a
crisis, it is essential to help them weigh the advantages and
risks of disclosure. In addition, for those who choose self-
disclosure to their families, it is important to provide follow
up support both for the individual who is coming out and for
his or her family. This may include a referral to gay-affirmative professional services, support groups, and religious counselors.

APPROPRIATE CRISIS INTERVENTION

In previous chapters Steele and Raider have described a 12-
stage crisis intervention model for use with students and their
families, and provided by school-based crisis workers. Regardless of their own sexual orientation, crisis workers,
teachers, counselors, and administrators can utilize this
model with sexual minority students and their families as
well. It is not necessary to be an "expert" on sexual minority
issues to be effective. Sexual minority youth come from every
imaginable type of background and family system: open,
closed, random, functional, dysfunctional, abusive, alcoholic,
divorced, single parent, large, small, ethnic minority, religious, nonreligious, and so forth. Therefore, as in any crisis
situation, an assessment of family characteristics is essential.
    People who are in crisis tend to be amenable to receiving
help (Rapoport, 1967), and the principles of crisis intervention theory apply regardless of the content of the presenting

problem. "The counselling and interpersonal skills that are effective with straight clients will be effective in work with homosexual clients, *if coupled with* a gay-affirmative attitude" (Schneider, 1988, p. 106).

Just what is a "gay-affirmative attitude"? Simply stated, it is a rational state of mind that allows the helper to approach a crisis in an unbiased fashion. To develop a gay-affirmative attitude, workers will need to understand and accept that:

- Homosexuality is neither a choice nor a particular lifestyle. Rather, "it is a naturally occurring variant in the expression of human sexuality" (DeCrescenzo, 1985 p. 134).
- Homosexuality is not an illness, nor a contagion, nor is it caused by poor family relations, seduction, or recruitment. The sexual orientation of gay and lesbian people does not pose a threat to others.
- The majority of sexual minority people are emotionally healthy and are capable of developing loving and caring relationships with family members, friends, and intimate partners (DeCrescenzo, 1985).
- Sexual minorities suffer from stigmatization and discrimination at all levels, which is based upon irrational fear and hatred. Sexual minority youth see this and take it to heart. This is the root cause for many self-destructive behaviors among gay and lesbian youth (Gibson, 1989).
- Family relations are just as important to sexual minorities as they are to heterosexuals. The sexual orientation of an individual does not make him or her a threat to the family—his or her own or anyone else's.
- Schools have a responsibility to provide a safe educational environment for *all* students.

There are several steps that workers can take to prepare themselves for dealing with sexual minorities and their families. These include: (1) examining your own beliefs about sexuality and homosexuality; (2) learning the facts about sexual minorities by reading, attending workshops and support group meetings, and getting to know homosexual people; (3) sharing what you learn with colleagues, friends, clients, and their families; (4) becoming a gay-affirmative role model, regardless of your own sexual orientation; (5) knowing your limits; and, (6) knowing the resources available for referrals. There is a growing body of literature, and a number of supportive organizations available to workers, sexual minority youth, and their families, several of which are listed at the end of this chapter.

Interventions with Students

Workers may encounter a range of crises related to sexual orientation including students who: are confused; have been "found out"; are considering "coming out"; or are feeling self-destructive over the awareness of their sexual orientation. The crisis intervention approach is appropriate for each of these conflicts. Though a complete discussion of detailed interventions is beyond the scope of this chapter, there are several basic guidelines that are common to each:

1. **Ask direct questions**. Sex and sexuality are always difficult for young people to discuss with adults. By asking direct questions in a nonjudgmental way, the worker helps to define the understanding of the crisis for both the worker and the client and to normalize the associated emotions. In order to allay fears about raising issues regarding sexuality, some youth counselors have found it useful to tell clients that they routinely ask about the sexual orientation of all clients.

2. **Assure confidentiality**. For adolescents who have sexual orientation concerns, this is absolutely critical. To inform their family before the student is prepared to deal with the possible reactions is to set the stage for additional crises, and serve to undermine any hope of establishing trust and rapport with the student. Even when there is a risk of suicide, you are only required to report the risk and not the detailed circumstances.

3. **Provide accurate information**. This implies knowing your limitations. Often, a crisis regarding sexual orientation is based upon either misinformation, a lack of information,

or both. This means that the worker must play a key role in providing or helping the student to obtain accurate information about homosexuality.

4. **Engage all available resources.** These include books, support groups, and therapists who employ a gay-affirmative approach. This also implies that workers must know their limitations and be willing to acknowledge them with the student or client. A useful strategy is to have the student report his or her findings back to the crisis worker after reading a book or attending a meeting or support group. Both parties will learn a great deal.

5. **Be available for follow up support.** This is particularly important when students decide or are forced to disclose their identity to the family. They will need to know that the worker is available both to themselves and to their family following the disclosure.

The worker can play a crucial role with sexual minority youth by facilitating the decision-making and planning process prior to disclosure to the family. Schneider (1988) provides a succinct description of these roles:

> Deciding whether or not to disclose involves: (a) weighing the risks and benefits, including parental response; and (b) examining the client's motivation [for disclosing].
> Planning for the disclosure involves considering: (a) the message [what and how it will be stated]; (b) method [letter, face-to-face, location, etc.]; (c) timing; (d) parent's probable reaction; and (e) [available] support.

For detailed discussions of each of these considerations the author highly recommends *Often Invisible: Counselling Gay and Lesbian Youth* (Schneider, 1988).

Interventions with Families

Successful crisis intervention requires the empowerment of those in crisis. However, the family's reaction to disclosure is not easily predictable and will depend upon their values and beliefs about homosexuality, as well as the nature of the family system. Some parents may feel relieved to have the truth out in the open, while others may feel as though the child has died. Concern for the child's future and a sense of guilt may become the dominant issues after initial disclosure. Others may wish to "change" the child and may become punitive or abusive. People such as Heather, David, Kevin, and Kirk have all faced the uncertainty of family reactions. David, Kevin, and Kirk all report that, after the initial shock and a somewhat lengthy period of adjustment, their families have begun to accept the reality and provide loving, caring support. Heather has developed a specific plan for disclosure and feels prepared this time to deal with any outcome.

In any case, it is important to understand that families go through stages in response to sexual orientation issues. Again, DeVine (1984) provides a model for understanding these stages. They are: (1) "subliminal awareness," or a sense that the child may have a same-gender orientation; (2) "impact," or the disclosure crisis; (3) "adjustment," which occurs immediately following the impact stage and is an effort to restabilize the family system; (4) "resolution," or the time when the family mourns its perceived losses and readjusts roles, rules, and expectations; and (5) "integration" of the focal member back into the system. Educators are most likely to encounter families of sexual minorities who are experiencing the first three stages, which incidentally are best treated from a crisis intervention perspective. The latter stages are best treated with gay-affirmative psychotherapy and support groups.

As DeVine (1984) points out, "When one selects to work with families where affectional preference is an issue, the role undertaken is that of guide" (p. 15). In order to effectively "guide" families through these stages of the disclosure crisis, workers will need to:

1. **Validate and normalize feelings**. This requires listening to and confronting the spoken and unspoken feelings experienced by family members. Gentle confrontation is useful in

defining perceptions of the crisis and accepting the associated emotions.

2. **Educate**. Parents need to know that homosexuality is a natural and healthy form of sexual expression and that they are not the "cause" of their child's orientation (Gibson, 1989). Family members also need to develop "constructive language" to cope with the crisis. It is usually helpful to provide parents with written materials on the subject and to arrange contact with supportive groups such as *Parents and Friends of Lesbians and Gays*. See the *Resources* section of this chapter for more information.

3. **Clarify homophobic responses**. This is also part of the educational process and will serve to prevent scapegoating of the focal member and identify misconceptions held by family members. Correcting these misconceptions can then become part of the problem-solving process.

4. **Assess the level of danger** (Steele & Raider, this volume). Keep in mind that sexual minority youth are at very high risk of suicide and physical abuse. When the potential for either is present, appropriate action must be taken. This may include removing the focal member, at least temporarily, from a potentially abusive or isolating environment.

5. **Strive for resolution and integration** (DeVine, 1984). Though adjustment is a normal stage, it is desirable to help the family grieve their losses, readjust the system, and integrate the focal member back into the family. This can be handled when structuring the intervention process by describing the stages of the disclosure crisis to the family and including resolution and integration as eventual goals of the intervention. It is best to inform the family that referral to a therapist or support group may be required, at some point, in order to accomplish these goals.

CONCLUSIONS

While searching for a way to conclude this chapter the author consulted a coworker who suggested providing some reassurances to those who will encounter sexual minority youth and their families.* When pressed for specifics, she replied, "Well, you don't have to be gay or lesbian yourself to help sexual minorities anymore than you have to have attempted suicide to help suicidal youth, nor do you have to come from an abusive family to help abused children and their families. Get the idea?" The point was well taken. Crisis intervention works with people who are in crisis, regardless of the content of the presenting problem.

The only additional requirements for those dealing with the problems experienced by gay and lesbian youth and their families are to: (1) acquire a gay-affirmative attitude by exploring personal beliefs, correcting misconceptions, and learning about the issues; and (2) achieve a level of comfort with the issues in order to maintain maximum effectiveness. This may not be possible for everyone. In this case, immediately involve a colleague or referral source who is comfortable dealing with sexual minority issues and who utilizes a gay-affirmative approach. In most cases, individuals in crisis will appreciate workers who are honest about their limitations much more than those who appear to be "in over their heads."

Finally, crisis intervention with the families of lesbian and gay youth is a short-term solution to a long-term problem. In order to reduce suicide, as well as the victimization of and discrimination against sexual minorities, educators and others must commit to dispelling the deeply ingrained misconceptions that perpetuate the irrational fears and hatred of homosexual people.

SUMMARY

The discovery that a child is lesbian or gay can cause a major crisis for families because they lack the appropriate roles,

*Sue Sells, M.A., M.P.H. (coworker) is a principal writer and editor of major grant proposals and educational publications for a large Community Mental Health Center. The author wishes to express his sincere appreciation for her input and critical feedback.

rules, and language to cope with the discovery. Families may respond to this discovery in a number of ways, and even highly functional families may be thrown into chaos. Sometimes families exclude the focal member through emotional distancing or physical removal in order to regain stability. This may place the nonheterosexual youth at a high risk of suicide or running away. Those from abusive and dysfunctional families are at an even higher risk.

Gay and lesbian people and their families make up almost one third of the entire U.S. population. Therefore, it is almost certain that educators will encounter sexual minority youth. Research has shown that sexual orientation is developed at an early age and is a natural occurrence. In addition, recent statistics show that many adolescents of all orientations are sexually active. This indicates that the school setting is an appropriate environment for addressing sexual minority issues. Since sexual minority youth are at a disproportionately high risk of suicide, violence, and discrimination on the basis of their sexual orientation, and since the school environment itself can contribute to increasing the risk, schools have crucial roles and responsibilities in providing appropriate crisis intervention and equal educational opportunities for sexual minorities and their families.

In order to do so, it is necessary for educators to dispel the misconceptions about homosexuality that perpetuate irrational fears and hatred. These include beliefs that homosexuality is a chosen lifestyle, contagious, an illness, a phase that will pass, and a threat to the institution of the family. Also, many believe that homosexuality should not be publicly disclosed. In fact: homosexuality occurs naturally to some degree in about 10% of the population; it is not a result of "seduction," "recruitment," or any other type of contagion; it is not the result of mental illness and therefore, it is not "curable"; it is distinct and separate from the normal adolescent "phases"; and it is in no way an indication that a person is anti-family or a threat to the family. Often, for gay and lesbian youth, the crisis is not a result of their homosexual orientation, but rather a result of the responses by others to their sexual orientation.

Regardless of their own sexual orientation, educators can effectively utilize the crisis intervention model with sexual minority youth and their families, as long as it is coupled with a "gay-affirmative" attitude. A gay-affirmative attitude is based upon fact rather than misconceptions, and allows crisis workers to approach sexual minority youth in an unbiased fashion. Workers can develop this kind of attitude by examining their own beliefs, learning and sharing the facts, becoming a gay-affirmative role model, and knowing the appropriate resources and referrals.

When providing crisis intervention for lesbian and gay youth there are several guidelines to be followed. These include: asking direct questions about sexuality; assuring confidentiality, especially when a young person is deciding whether or not to tell the family; providing accurate information; engaging all available resources, such as gay-affirmative books, therapists, and support groups; and being available for follow-up support, particularly after disclosure to the family. The worker can be very helpful in facilitating the young person's decision whether or not to tell his or her family, and how to tell them when the time comes.

Families go through definable stages when they discover the homosexual orientation of a member. School crisis workers can be very helpful, particularly during the initial or crisis stages. The role of the worker is to "guide" the family through the stages by validating and normalizing their feelings, educating them to the facts and dispelling the misconceptions that serve to place "blame" on the family, clarifying homophobic responses, assessing the danger to the focal member, and setting goals to resolve the crisis and integrate the focal member back into the family.

The sexual orientation of the helper is irrelevant as long as the helper is able to achieve a gay-affirmative attitude and a high enough level of comfort with sexual minority issues to be effective. Since this may not be possible for everyone, appropriate referrals are crucial, and most likely will be appreciated by those in crisis. In addition to providing appropriate crisis intervention, schools need to address the environmental issues and discrimination that put sexual minority youth at a disproportionately high risk of suicide, verbal abuse, and physical assault.

REFERENCES

Alcohol, Drug Abuse, and Mental Health Administration. (1989). *Report of the Secretary's Task Force on Youth Suicide* (Vols. 1-4). Washington, DC: Superintendent of Documents, U.S. Government Printing Office.

American Psychiatric Association. (1987). *Diagnostic and statistical manual of mental disorders* (3rd ed.-revised [DSM-III-R]). Washington, DC: Author.

Bell, A. P., & Weinberg, M. S. (1978). *Homosexualities: A study of diversity among men and women.* New York: Simon and Schuster.

Bell, A. P., Weinberg, M. S., & Hammersmith, S. K. (1981). *Sexual preference: Its development in men and women.* Bloomington: Indiana University Press.

Bohn, T. R. (1983). *Violence against gay men and lesbians: Empirical research on trends in homophobic violence.* Unpublished master's thesis, School of Social Welfare, State University of New York at Stony Brook.

Bohn, T. R. (1984). Homophobic violence: Implications for social work practice. In R. Schoenberg, R. S. Goldberg, with D. A. Shore (Eds.), *With compassion toward some: Homosexuality and social work in America.* New York: Harrington Park Press.

Boswell, J. (1980). *Christianity, social tolerance, and homosexuality.* Chicago: University of Chicago Press.

Bozett, F. W. (1989). Preface. In F. W. Bozett (Ed.), *Homosexuality and the family* (pp. xi-xiv). New York: Harrington Park Press.

Burgess, A. W., Groth, A. N., Holmstrom, L. L., & Sgroi, S. M. (1978). *Sexual assault of children and adolescents.* Lexington, MA: D. C. Heath.

Centers for Disease Control (1985). *Statistical report on suicide.* Atlanta: Author.

Clark, D. (1987). *The new loving someone gay: Revised and updated.* Berkeley, CA: Celestial Arts.

Cook, A. T. (1988). *And God loves each one: A resource for dialogue about the church and homosexuality.* Washington, DC: Reconciling Congregation Program.

Davies, P. (Ed.). (1980). *The American heritage dictionary of the English language.* New York: Dell Publishing.

DeCrescenzo, T. A. (1985). Homophobia: A study of the attitudes of mental health professionals toward homosexuality. In R. Schoenberg, R. S. Goldberg, with D. A. Shore (Eds.), *With compassion toward some: Homosexuality and social work in America* (pp. 115-136). New York: Harrington Park Press.

DeFrancis, V. (1966). *Protecting the child victim of sex crimes committed by adults.* Denver: American Humane Association.

DeVine, J. L. (1984). A systematic inspection of affectional preference orientation and the family of origin. In R. Schoenberg, R. S. Goldberg, with D. A. Shore (Eds.), *With compassion toward some: Homosexuality and social work in America* (pp. 9-17). New York: Harrington Park Press.

Federal Bureau of Investigation. (1986). *Uniform crime reports, 1986: Crime in the United States.* Washington, DC: U.S. Department of Justice.

Freedman, M. (1975). Stimulus-response: Homosexuals may be healthier than straights. *Psychology Today, 8*(10), 28-32.

Freud, S. (1903). Quoted in *Die Ziet,* Vienna, October 27, 1903, 5.

Gibson, P. (1989). Gay male and lesbian youth suicide. In Alcohol, Drug Abuse, and Mental Health Administration, *Report of the Secretary's Task Force on Youth Suicide* (Vol. 3: Prevention and interventions in youth suicide, pp. 110-142). DHHS Pub. No. (AD)89-1623. Washington, DC: Superintendent of Documents, U.S. Government Printing Office.

Gonsiorek, J. C. (1982). Results of psychological testing on homosexual populations. In W. Paul, J. D. Weinrich, J. C. Gonsiorek, & M. E. Hotvedt (Eds.), *Homosexuality: Social, psychological and biological issues* (pp. 71-80). Beverly Hills, CA: Sage Publications.

Griffin, C. W., Wirth, M. J., & Wirth, A. G. (1986). *Beyond acceptance: Parents of lesbian and gays talk about their experiences.* Englewood Cliffs, NJ: Prentice-Hall.

Groth, A. N., & Birnbaum, H. J. (1978). Adult sexual orientation and attraction to underage children. *Archives of Sexual Behavior, 7,* 175-181.

Hiltner, S. (1980). Homosexuality and the churches. In J. Marmor (Ed.), *Homosexual behavior*, (pp. 219-231). New York: Basic Books.

Hooker, E. A. (1957). The adjustment of the male overt homosexual. *Journal of Protective Techniques, 21*(1), 17-31.

House Select Committee on Children, Youth and Families. (1987). *Fact sheet: AIDS and teenagers*. Washington, DC: U.S. Government Printing Office.

Isay, R. A. (1989). *Being homosexual: Gay men and their development*. New York: Farrar Straus Giroux.

Kempe, R. S., & Kempe, C. S. (1984). *The common secret: Sexual abuse of children and adolescents*. New York: W. H. Freeman.

Kinsey, A. C., Pomeroy, W. B., & Martin, C. E. (1948). *Sexual behavior in the human male*. Philadelphia: W. B. Saunders.

Kinsey, A. C., Pomeroy, W. B., Martin, C. E., & Gebhard, P. H. (1953). *Sexual behavior in the human female*. Philadelphia: W. B. Saunders.

Lee, J. A. (1977). Going public: A study in the sociology of homosexual liberation. *Journal of Homosexuality, 3,* 49-78.

Malyon, A. K. (1982). Psychotherapeutic implications of internalized homophobia in gay men. In J. C. Gonsiorek (Ed.), *A guide to psychotherapy with gay and lesbian clients* (pp. 59-69). New York: Harrington Park Press.

Martin, A. D. (1984). The perennial canaanites: The sin of homosexuality. *Et Cetera, 41,* 340-361.

Martin, A. D., & Hetrick, E. S. (1988). The stigmatization of the gay and lesbian adolescent. *Journal of Homosexuality, 15*(1/2), 163-183.

McDonald, G. (1982). Individual differences in the coming-out process for gay men: Implications for theoretical models. *Journal of Homosexuality, 8,* 47-60.

McNeill, J. (1988). *The church and homosexuality* (3rd ed., updated and expanded). Boston: Beacon Press.

Norton, J. L. (1976, March). The homosexual and counseling. *Personnel and Guidance Journal, 54,* 374-377.

Parris, F. (1985, May 17). Some die young. *Washington Blade,* 3-128.

Pomeroy, W. B. (1972). *Dr. Kinsey and the Institute for Sex Research*. New York: Harper & Row.

Rapoport, L. (1967, March). Crisis oriented short term casework. *Social Service Review,* 38-41.

Schneider, M. S. (1988). *Often invisible: Counselling gay & lesbian youth.* Toronto: Central Toronto Youth Services.

Star, B. (1979). Research perspectives on the impact of sexual abuse. In *Proceedings of the Fourth National Conference on child abuse and neglect* (pp. 124–127). Washington, DC: U.S. Department of Health, Education, and Welfare.

Strommen, E. F. (1990). Hidden branches and growing pains: Homosexuality and the family tree. In F. W. Bozett & M. B. Sussman (Eds.), *Homosexuality and family relations.* New York: Harrington Park Press.

Tartagni, D. (1978). Counseling gays in a school setting. *School Counselor, 26,* 26–32.

Woodman, N. J. (1985). Parents of lesbians and gays: Concerns and intervention. In H. Hidalgo, T. L. Peterson, & N. J. Woodman (Eds.), *Lesbian and gay issues: A resource manual for social workers* (pp. 21–32). Silver Springs, MD: National Association of Social Workers.

Zeh, J. (1989). Sullivan backs Dannemeyer's attack on youth suicide report. *Gay Community News, 17*(8), 3.

Zelnick, M., & Shah, F. (1983). First intercourse among young Americans. *Family Planning Perspectives, 15*(2), 64–70.

ADDITIONAL READING

Back, G. G. (1985). *Are you still my mother? Are you still my family?* New York: Warner Books.

Berzon, B. (1988). *Permanent partners: Building gay & lesbian relationships that last.* New York: E. P. Dutton.

Dilley, J. W., Pies, C., & Helquist, M. (Eds.). (1989). *Face to face: A guide to AIDS counseling.* Berkeley, CA: Celestial Arts.

Fairchild, B., & Hayward, N. (1989). *Now that you know: What every parent should know about homosexuality.* San Diego: Harcourt Brace Jovanovich.

Fierstein, H. (1978). *Torch song trilogy.* New York: Signet.

Heron, A. (Ed.). (1983). *One teenager in 10: Writings by gay and lesbian youth.* Boston: Alyson Publications.

Kain, C. (Ed.). (1989). *No longer immune: A counselor's guide to AIDS.* Alexandria, VA: American Association for Counseling and Development.

McWhirter, D. P., & Mattison, A. M. (1984). *The male couple: How relationships develop.* Englewood Cliffs, NJ: Prentice-Hall.
Rofes, E. E. (1983). *I thought people like that killed themselves: Lesbians, gay men and suicide.* San Francisco: Grey Fox Press.

RESOURCES

For young people with concerns about sexual orientation:
I.Y.G. Youth Hotline
P.O. Box 20716
Indianapolis, IN 46220
(800) 347-TEEN 7 P.M.—12 A.M. (Central time), Friday and Saturday.
(317) 635-TEEN in Indianapolis.

For families dealing with the crisis of discovering and accepting the sexual orientation of a member:
P-FLAG, Family and Chapter Support Office
P.O. Box 27605
Washington, D.C. 20038-7605
(202) 638-4200

Listening, Learning, Loving: Parents of Lesbians and Gays (30-minute video). Available from:
Parent's FLAG–Detroit
P.O. Box 145
Farmington, MI 48332
(313) 478-8408.

For those with religious concerns:
And God Loves Each One: A Resource for Dialogue about the Church and Homosexuality (booklet). Available from:
Reconciling Congregation Program
P.O. Box 23636
Washington, D.C. 20026

For those concerned about AIDS and sexually transmitted diseases:
National AIDS Hotline

(800) 342-AIDS, 24 hours daily.
(800) 344-7432 (Spanish speaking), 8 A.M.—2 A.M. (Eastern time),
daily.
(800) 243-7889 (TTY/TDD), 10 A.M.—10 P.M. (Eastern time), daily.

National STD Hotline
(800) 227-8922, 8 A.M.—11 P.M. (Eastern time), Monday—Friday.

**Professional educational associations that have adopted policies of
nondiscrimination on the basis of sexual orientation:**
American Federation of Teachers (AFT)
Association of Supervision and Curriculum Development (ASCD)
National Educational Association (NEA)

Appendix:
Guides and Tools for
the Stages of Intervention

STAGE ONE: Structuring the Interview Process

Structuring Statements

• We are going to approach this as a crisis situation and as such you can expect to have some resolution in 4-6 weeks.

• There are two possible outcomes of this process. The situation may be resolved. If the situation cannot be changed, you will have regained control so that the situation is no longer the threat to you it is now. The other possibility is that we will be unable to resolve this crisis. However, we will be better able to identify what is actually causing it and what is needed to resolve it. So we can, if necessary, bring in or refer you to the appropriate resource so that it can be resolved in the shortest period possible.

• We will meet as often as is necessary during the next 4-6 weeks, and as quickly as possible should you request an unscheduled visit. Difficulties are much easier to resolve when they arise, as opposed to having them go on for several days before getting to them.

• Some sessions may last longer than others. We will meet as long as is necessary to resolve the particular issue we are dealing with.

• Initially I will have many questions to ask all of you. The more information you can provide the easier it becomes for us to arrive at a solution.

• You may also ask me questions, and if you do I will be as direct as I can be and give you my honest opinions.

• If I do not have the answers to your questions I will tell you, and then find the answers by the next session, or while you wait if it is an urgent situation.

• You need to understand how I approach a family in crisis. Rarely does any one family member have the sole burden of the problem. A family is like any other organization, team, or group of people who work together. If one of the members is not fulfilling his or her role, living up to expectations and obligations, of failing to perform his or her duties, the entire organization, team, group, or family is put in crisis. Whenever one member of a family changes, or a person's condition changes, the entire family faces new challenges, changes, and choices.

• We will therefore work on not blaming any one person in this family for what is occurring, and look both at the problem that this crisis has created for each of you and at the ways that you as a family can pool your resources, learn from this crisis, and get back on track.

• I will not ask you to try any solution without first looking at what the possible consequences might be. If you are uncomfortable with the proposed solution we will simply work together to find another.

• Let me give you a warning. Some of our solutions may sound very good here in the office but fail miserably when you try to implement them. This does not mean that either you or I have failed, but only that the solution simply was not the best solution at this time. In that situation we just move to our next alternative.

• Sometimes in this process the crisis seems to get worse not better. This happens because as we begin to take a look at an issue other problems begin to emerge. This is also the time when families tend to give up. Keep in mind that when additional problems begin to emerge it means that we are making progress and clarifying how this crisis has effected each and every one of you. When we know this it is much easier to make decisions as to how best to resolve the crisis. So when things seem to be getting worse, let me know, but also remember that it is a sign of progress. Also, keep in mind that by the end of the four to six week period you will know much more about your situation, including what works, what doesn't work, and what you will need to do to maintain any progress we have made.

• Should a serious crisis arise and you feel you need assistance outside of our school hours I want to give you several numbers that you can call to get immediate assistance with that one crisis. I encourage you to call should this happen, and to call me the next morning so that we can be sure to resolve the situation.

• Before we conclude our session today I'm going to introduce you to some of my colleagues (team members). This is for your benefit. If for some reason I am not available when you need to meet with me, one of my colleagues will be able to help out. I will keep them apprised of our sessions so that they can be of help to me as well as to you should you need immediate attention. No one else will know of your situation. All information will be kept confidential and not be placed in your son's/daughter's public file.

• Also, before we conclude today you will know exactly what will be taking place during the next few days. This we will agree on together.

• I want you to feel free to let me know when you think I am way off base. I'm sure I may say some things that are, but if you do not let me know I will proceed on the basis that I am correct. This will not be helpful for either of us.

• Finally, there are some ground rules for our sessions. Because we are dealing with a crisis and you have fears about the worst that can happen, some of our sessions may become very emotional. I must have your agreement on the following conditions:

1. There will be no physical contact, like hitting, shoving, or punching.
2. Initially yelling may be unavoidable, but when I ask everyone to stop I expect you to so that we can all collect our thoughts.
3. Should you want to discontinue counseling I ask that you let me know here in my office so that I can provide you with a summary of my thoughts as to what might be helpful for you in the future.
4. Finally, I want you to know that should you feel like discontinuing counseling because you simply are not satisfied or feel that we do not understand one another, tell me this. I will not take offense, and I will give you several referrals. Counseling is no different than seeking the services of a physician. If you don't like or trust a physician you find one that you can trust.

• I know that I have given you a lot to think about, but I want you to know how this process works, what you can expect from me, and what I expect from you. Are there any questions? If not, how about we start by one of you telling me more about what has been happening.

STAGE TWO: Questions for Defining Family's Understanding of Their Crisis*

1. We were not aware that any problems existed before today. Perhaps there were problems, but we did not recognize them, so what brought you here today as opposed to a week ago?
2. Do you have any ideas about what started this?
3. What were your initial reactions and what are your reactions, thoughts, and concerns now?
4. Why do you think that this crisis is not going away?
5. What have you tried to do?

*Refer to Chapter 6 for explanations of each question.

6. How does it leave you feeling?

7. What does it make you feel like doing?

8. Is there anyone else involved—relatives, friends?

9. What makes this situation more difficult than others that you have faced?

10. Do you think that this is an uncommon situation for families? Do you feel that you have handled it like most families would? (explain)

11. Who or what is hurting you the most right now?

STAGE THREE: Defining the Intervenor's Understanding of the Crisis*

1. What unexpected, unwanted, unfamiliar, or new situation or condition has occurred in the past two weeks?

2. Has anything new, unfamiliar, unwanted, or unexpected happened to anyone else you know?

3. Have you ever felt like this before? If so when, and what was happening?

4. What other problems has this created for you?

5. Have there been any changes because of this situation?

6. What positive changes have occurred in the past several weeks?

STAGE FOUR: Questions for Determining the Type of Family System**

1. Rule: How and who makes the rules in your home?

2. Focus: How do you want others to see your family?

3. Affection: In what ways do you usually express affection?

4. Goal: What is the major goal your family strives to achieve and maintain?

*Refer to Chapter 6 for explanations of each question.

**Refer to Chapter 7 for explanations of each question.

TABLE A.1. Stage Four: Determining Family System Type (Overview of Family System Characteristics)

Area of assessment	Type		
	Closed	Open	Random
1. Rule:	Authoritarian	Participatory	Random, anybody
2. Focus:	Family image of unity even if unity does not exist	Individual needs and family unity	Individual desires chosen over family unity
3. Affection: (Emotional bondings)	Covert	Overt	Overt and covert
4. Goal:	Stability	Flexibility	Spontaneity, exploration tolerated–encouraged
5. Ambiguity:	Not tolerated	Tolerated until clarity reached	Tolerated–encouraged
6. Conflict:	Not tolerated	Seen as healthy process	Inconsistent
7. Decision making:	Autocratic	Family participation	Individualistic
8. Information processing:	One-way (top-down)	Three-way (top-down, down-up, and across)	Random, inconsistent
9. Communication:	Secretive, restrictive pattern	Open, sharing, listening, negotiating patterns	Informal, from closed to open pattern
10. In a crisis:	Rigid, unyielding; creates greater vulnerability and potential for further deterioration	Yielding, flexible; open to help minimizing vulnerability and risk of continued deterioration	Lacks sufficient consistency; leaves it vulnerable but not at as great a risk as the closed system due to its tolerance for ambiguity

5. Ambiguity: Do you like change?
6. Conflict: How do you manage conflict?
7. Decision making: When there is a major decision to be made how is it made and who makes it?
8. Information process: How does information usually get passed on in your family?
9. Communication: Would you say that everybody knows everyone else's business in your family or do you tend to believe that not everyone needs to know or should know everyone's business?
10. In a crisis: The previous nine questions will reveal the patterns reflected in each of the system descriptions in this category (see Table 2.1).

STAGE FIVE

Part I: Questions for Determining Boundary Inhibitors and/or Strengths*

1. How do you feel about getting help?
2. How do you feel about sharing your difficulties with an outsider?
3. How do you feel about paying for this service?
4. Do you believe talking really helps?
5. Do you believe that I should be talking to the entire family about this problem or just to the person(s) who seem to have the major problem?

If we have adequately explained the differences between the systems, you will know that closed systems will respond negatively to these questions. They will not be comfortable asking for help, bringing in an outsider, or sharing their difficulties with extended family members or even with other immediate family members. They will begrudge paying for such services and will not like the idea of trying to bring things out into the open. They will not believe in the family approach, but rather

*Refer to Chapter 7 for explanation.

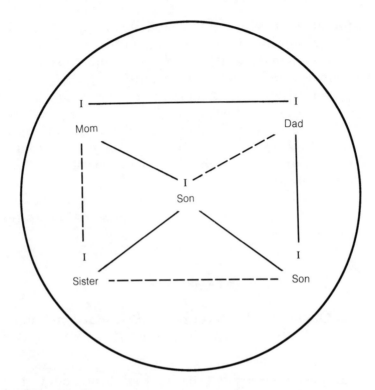

FIGURE A.1. Subsystem relationships. Solid lines are strong relationships. Broken lines are weak relationships.

in addressing the person (often the scapegoat) who is exhibiting the most problematic behavior.

Part II: Determining Subsystem Inhibitors or Strengths*

Step 1: Make and pass out two copies of Figure A.1 to each of the family members (attached).

*This exercise may meet with defensiveness because of the fear members may have of one another. If nothing else, the way individual members portray their relationships can be compared to the nature of the interactions they reveal during the intervention process, and then addressed as incongruities arise.

Step 2: Have family correct the individual identities (i.e., two daughters, but only one son). Also, have them fill in the names of children.

Step 3: Have the family place the number "1" in the upper right hand corner of the first diagram. Explain that this drawing pictures how things were before the crisis, and then instruct each member to: a) draw a circle around who he or she is in the drawing; b) draw a solid line from themselves to other member(s) they feel the closest to; and c) a dotted line to the member(s) they do not feel as close to.

Step 4: Have family members place the number "2" in upper right hand corner of the second drawing. Explain that this drawing pictures how things have been since the crisis (trouble) and then have them complete the "a," "b," and "c" process in step three.

Step 5: Place drawing number "1" on the board for all to see. Process with them their responses, surprises, agreements, and questions as to why each felt close to the person(s) they designated.

Step 6: Place drawing number "2" on the board for all to see. Process (using additional questions) what has changed about the individuals who were connected with a solid line in Drawing "1" and broken line in Diagram "2."

It is helpful to mention that rarely do relationships stay the same in the face of a crisis. When the crisis ends the relationships may return to what they were before or change, and may improve or deteriorate. Indicate that if a relationship does deteriorate you will be available to help them.

Part III: Family Processes Strength-Weakness Guide

Using the scale below and the information and family interaction observed during the first four stages, rate the strength or weakness of the family processes. Weak represents a nonfunctional or problematic process. Strong represents a supportive functional process. (See Chapter 7 for explanations of the processes.)

Circle the appropriate rating.	Weak		Moderate		Strong
Emotional bonding	1	2	3	4	5
Decision making	1	2	3	4	5
Information processing	1	2	3	4	5
Conflict resolution	1	2	3	4	5
Communication	1	2	3	4	5

STAGE SIX:

Part I: Assessing the Level of Danger

The following assessment tools are only guides to help alert you to a number of known risk factors in a family.

A list of known risk factors is presented. Their presence in any system has the potential for increasing the level of danger. The more factors present, the higher the risk potential. Keep in mind, however, the family's generational history, cultural and ethnic backgrounds, financial status, and so on. What may be a significantly high risk factor for one family may not be for another.

The absence of risk factors does not necessarily indicate that there is no danger present. This is the reason that a second consultation is necessary in any crisis.

The presence of any one risk factor may in and of itself reflect a potentially lethal situation that requires further exploration. The information and tools provided in this section, therefore, must be viewed in the context of what you know about the family and its members. Also, keep in mind that it is always advisable to consult with colleagues about your assessment of the level of danger prior to determining your intervention strategy and/or concluding the interview.

Part II: Questions That Can Help Determine The Potential for Danger (Self or Others)

- Is there a history of similar behavior?
- Has there been a history of help, but has this been seen as a negative experience?

- Has there been a history or series of losses preceding this particular crisis?
- Has there been a history of poor impulse control?
- Has there been a history of chaos in the family?
- Does the family find it difficult to change, even in the face of repeated problems?
- Has there been a history of depression in one of the parents and/or the single parent?
- Is there a current drug or substance abuse problem?
- Is there a history of academic difficulties?
- Is the youth unable to communicate his or her feelings and thoughts?
- Is there an inability to entertain recommendations or a "yes but" response to recommendations and explanations?
- Is there a refusal to accept recommendations?
- Is there an inability to compliment oneself or identify one's strengths?
- Is there an inability to perceive others as not only caring but helpful?
- Is there an inability to engage in the problem-solving process?

Part III: Maladaptive Responses That Can Increase Risk Factors

The following is a list of maladaptive family responses when their members are faced with a crisis. The opposite of each of these responses becomes an adaptive response. These responses include both the family system responses and family processes.

1. Emotionally detached, cold, aloof
2. Emotionally explosive, unpredictable and/or helpless and hopeless
3. Unwillingness to communicate
4. Unwillingness to ask for or accept help
5. Closed to new ways of coping
6. Absence of family involvement in decision making
7. Inability to alter roles, responsibilities, or expectations during a crisis

8. Denial, withdrawal, or avoidance of the inherent conflicts within a crisis
9. Lack of direction, guidance, or support among the
   members
10. Scapegoating, blaming
11. Substance abuse, including alcohol

Additional Factors Related to Suicide

When someone gives away prized possessions he or she may
have decided to end his or her life, or may be simply be trying
to make a friend. Such behaviors or warning signs, however,
can only tell us that something is different. An inability to
concentrate could be due to a physical illness or stress, or to
the depression associated with suicidal thinking. The only
way to know for sure whether or not someone is thinking
about suicide is to ask the person when you observe behavior
that concerns you. Be aware that when assessing risk, the
higher the number of risk factors present the higher the risk.
This does not mean, however, that if only a few of the risk
factors are present there is little likelihood for an attempt.
Someone who has no plan, only an ideation, but has a history
of poor impulse control, could be considered high risk. We
reiterate the importance of a second opinion by another
member of your crisis team and/or by an outside referral
source. The determination of risk, and of the course of any
subsequent interventions, should not be the responsibility of
one person. The following factors are frequently part of tools
used to assess suicide lethality.

Has a specific plan: method is available; when, where is
   determined
Alcohol/substance ingested or known problem
Previous suicide attempt (the more lethal the attempt, the
   higher the risk)
Poor impulse control
Recent attempt/completion by a significant other
Loss of a significant other
Family history of suicide

Chronic depression of parent
Closed family characteristics
Expressed sense of hopelessness
Constricted thinking (always–never, either–or response to situation)
Poor problem-solving skills
Poor communication skills
History of physical/sexual victimization
Sexual preference issue
Unable to compliment self
Refuses "no suicide" contact or recommendations
Expressed guilt/shame
Psychomotor retardation/agitation
Aggressive behavior
Diminished socialization
Change in attitude toward school/future
Sleeping/eating disturbances
Loss of motivation
Fatigue
Inability to concentrate
Somatic complaints

Additional Factors Related to Violence

There are no reliable predictors of violence. However, a profile of a potentially violent individual can be constructed by taking into account the following factors:

Social History

- Previous history of violent behavior, especially if weapons were used or there is a criminal record of violence such as assault, armed robbery, etc.
- Poor record of employment or school performance
- History of antisocial behavior, such as a lack of conscience or remorse
- Social isolation and/or lack of social supports

Family

- History of violence in the family
- Victim of early physical or sexual abuse
- Early loss or separation from a parent
- Recent traumatic loss (e.g., grief stricken family member, lover, etc.)

Personality and Psychological Factors

- Poor problem-solving or coping skills
- Poor impulse control or a history of aggressive outbursts
- Dependency or counter-dependency, especially when faced with real or perceived rejection (e.g., Hyper-masculine male, domestic violence perpetrator, etc.)
- Obsession with an unavailable person or object
- Homosexual panic or obsessive homophobia, particularly when resulting from a recent encounter or assault
- Alcohol or substance abuse, especially if ingested today
- History of suicide attempts
- Psychotic behavior (hallucinations, delusions, mania, etc.)
- Poor object-relations or ego functions (e.g., borderline personality disorder)
- Organic brain syndrome, dementia (e.g., confused, disoriented, etc.)

Current Behavior

- Loss of power (real or perceived)
- Stated fear of losing control
- Agitated or labile
- Extreme withdrawal
- Lack of personal physical boundaries (self and/or others)
- Inappropriate emotional intensity
- Intense, unbroken glares (the "scary stare")
- Threats (the more irrational, the greater the risk)
- Plans (the more specific and the more available the method, the greater the risk)
- Intuitive fear by others (staff, other clients, etc.)

Though not absolute, a *a history of violence* and/or an *intuitive fear by others* are the most reliable predictors of the potential for violence.

STAGE SEVEN: Presenting a Different Understanding of the Crisis

1. Normalize the situation
2. Provide an acceptable explanation for the cause of their reactions. The focus of the explanation is their response to loss (see Figure 8.1, circle of loss and fear).

STAGE EIGHT: Identification, Acceptance, and Management of Feelings

1. Use Figure 8.1 to help family members identify the most unwanted or threatening feelings.
2. Reach a consensus as to which feeling is presenting the most difficulties.
3. Ask what, at its worst, this feeling makes them want to do, and then clarify for them that feelings do not need to be acted upon.

STAGE NINE: Engaging the Family in the Problem-Solving Process

1. Educate the family to the benefits of the problem-solving process. See Chapter 9 for model statements to present to the family.
2. Present the problem-solving chart (Figure 9.1) and review with the family.

STAGES TEN AND ELEVEN:
Identification and Selection of Problem;
Setting Time Tables

1. Review Chapter 9 for discussion of these stages. Figure 9.1 summarizes the problem-solving process.

STAGE TWELVE: Reassessing the Family Status

1. Ask the family if they feel more hopeful and in control than at the beginning of the intervention.
2. Reassess the appropriateness of scheduling another session, making a referral or taking emergency measures.

Index

Self-defeating behavior, 8–9, 110
Self-destructive behavior, 91, 92, 104
Self-help group, homicide, 136–137
Self-mutilation, 152
Separation, 36
Sexual abuse, 148
Sexual assault, 62
Sexually transmitted diseases, 165, 191–192
Sexual-minority youth, 161–187
  coming out to family, 161–163, 177, 182, 185
  common misconceptions about homosexuality, 167–178
  crisis intervention, 178–183, 186
  definition, 162, 163
  prevalence, 164–165, 185
  rejection, 163, 169, 173
  resources, listed, 191–192
  schools, 164–167, 179
  suicide, 165–167, 178, 184
  taboos against, 162
  targets of assaults, 165, 166, 173, 184
Sexual precocity, 4
Sexual preference, 113
Sexual promiscuity, 151
Sex, unsafe, 91
Shame-based family system, 148–149, 158–159
Single-parent households, 4, 36
  and chemical dependency, 153
Skill rehearsal, 106
Sleep disturbance, child witness to parent's murder, 134
Social activity and coping, 37–38
Social history, danger assessment (stage six), 205
Social learning theory, 149–150
Social reinforcement, chemical dependency, 149–151
Social withdrawal, 152
Solutions, identification and selection (ten), 50, 108, 110–111, 208
Stages, twelve stages, of crisis intervention, 43–52

Stealing, 91
Step-families, 5
Stigma after suicide, 129
Subsystems, family system, 47, 89–90, 200–201
Suicide, 4, 5, 8, 11, 60, 63, 76, 78, 100, 113, 151
  case report, contagion effect, 120–128
  conspiracy of silence, 126–127
  crisis team, 122
  depression, 124, 125
  suicidal ideation, 124, 125
  teaching staff, 127
  triage, 122–123
  and chemical dependency, 146
  danger, assessment (stage six), 91, 93, 204–205
  families and grief, 128–132
  and helplessness, 129–130
  sexual-minority youth, 165–166, 167, 178, 184
Suicide: After a Suicide What Can We Do?, 130

Teaching staff, teen suicide, 127
Team approach, 58
They Help Each Other Spiritually (THEOS), 137
Time-table for problem-solving (stage eleven), 50–51, 112, 208
Triage, teen suicide, 122–123
Truancy, 152

Unemployment, 79

Validation, feelings of families of gay youth, 182–183, 198
Violence, 5, 6, 38, 76, 113
  assessment, 91, 205, 207
  of suicide, 129
Violent death, 62

Witness to parents' murder, 134–137
Work activity, compulsive, 148
Working parents, 5